Christian Joffroy

Antiestrogens induce immunosuppression

Christian Joffroy

Antiestrogens induce immunosuppression

Tamoxifen and Fulvestrant lead to TGFß-mediated immunosuppression in breast cancer

Südwestdeutscher Verlag für Hochschulschriften

Impressum/Imprint (nur für Deutschland/ only for Germany)

Bibliografische Information der Deutschen Nationalbibliothek: Die Deutsche Nationalbibliothek verzeichnet diese Publikation in der Deutschen Nationalbibliografie; detaillierte bibliografische Daten sind im Internet über http://dnb.d-nb.de abrufbar.

Alle in diesem Buch genannten Marken und Produktnamen unterliegen warenzeichen-, marken- oder patentrechtlichem Schutz bzw. sind Warenzeichen oder eingetragene Warenzeichen der jeweiligen Inhaber. Die Wiedergabe von Marken, Produktnamen, Gebrauchsnamen, Handelsnamen, Warenbezeichnungen u.s.w. in diesem Werk berechtigt auch ohne besondere Kennzeichnung nicht zu der Annahme, dass solche Namen im Sinne der Warenzeichen- und Markenschutzgesetzgebung als frei zu betrachten wären und daher von jedermann benutzt werden dürften.

Verlag: Südwestdeutscher Verlag für Hochschulschriften Aktiengesellschaft & Co. KG
Dudweiler Landstr. 99, 66123 Saarbrücken, Deutschland
Telefon +49 681 37 20 271-1, Telefax +49 681 37 20 271-0
Email: info@svh-verlag.de
Zugl.: Stuttgart, Universität, Diss., 2006

Herstellung in Deutschland:
Schaltungsdienst Lange o.H.G., Berlin
Books on Demand GmbH, Norderstedt
Reha GmbH, Saarbrücken
Amazon Distribution GmbH, Leipzig
ISBN: 978-3-8381-1671-6

Imprint (only for USA, GB)

Bibliographic information published by the Deutsche Nationalbibliothek: The Deutsche Nationalbibliothek lists this publication in the Deutsche Nationalbibliografie; detailed bibliographic data are available in the Internet at http://dnb.d-nb.de.

Any brand names and product names mentioned in this book are subject to trademark, brand or patent protection and are trademarks or registered trademarks of their respective holders. The use of brand names, product names, common names, trade names, product descriptions etc. even without a particular marking in this works is in no way to be construed to mean that such names may be regarded as unrestricted in respect of trademark and brand protection legislation and could thus be used by anyone.

Publisher: Südwestdeutscher Verlag für Hochschulschriften Aktiengesellschaft & Co. KG
Dudweiler Landstr. 99, 66123 Saarbrücken, Germany
Phone +49 681 37 20 271-1, Fax +49 681 37 20 271-0
Email: info@svh-verlag.de

Printed in the U.S.A.
Printed in the U.K. by (see last page)
ISBN: 978-3-8381-1671-6

TABLE OF CONTENTS

1 LIST OF ABBREVIATIONS

°C	degree celsius
μl	microliter
AE	antiestrogens
ag	attogram
APC	antigen presenting cells
APS	ammonium persulfate
as	antisense
bp	base pair
BrdU	5 bromodeoxyuridine
BSA	bovine serum albumin
CCS	charcoal-stripped FCS
cDNA	complementary DNA
cntr	control
CTL	cytotoxic T lymphocytes
DC	dendritic cells
DMEM	Dulbecco's modified eagle medium
DMSO	dimethylsulfoxide
DNA	deoxyribonucleic acid
dNTP	deoxyribonucleotide triphosphate
EBCTCG	early breast cancer trialists collaborative group
EDTA	ethylenediaminetetraacetic acid
EGTA	ethylene glycol tetraacetic acid
ELISA	enzyme-linked immunosorbent assay
EMT	epithelial-mesenchymal transition
EpCAM	epithelial cell adhesion molecule
ER	estrogen receptor
ERE	estrogen response element
et al.	et aliter
F	Farad
FasL	Fas ligand
FCS	fetal calf serum
fg	femtogram

Fig	figure
Foxp3	forkhead box P3
G418	geneticin-disulphate
GUS	ß-glucuronidase
GzmB	granzyme B
h	hour
HCl	hydrochloric acid
HRP	horseradish peroxidase
ICI	ICI 182.780 (Fulvestrant)
IFNγ	Interferon gamma
IL-2	interleukin-2
kDa	kilodalton
LDH	lactate dehydrogenase
MACS	magnetic cell sorting
MHC	major histocompatibility complex
min	minute
ml	milliliter
MLTR	mixed lymphocyte tumor reaction
mM	micromolar
mRNA	messenger ribonucleic acid
NaCl	sodium chloride
NK cells	natural killer cells
OHT	4-hydroxytamoxifen
PBMC	peripheral blood mononuclear cells
PBS	phosphate buffered saline
PCR	polymerase chain reaction
PMSF	phenylmethylsulfonyl fluoride
PRF1	perforin
qRT-PCR	quantitative real time PCR
RNA	ribonucleic acid
rpm	rounds per minute
RT	reverse transcription
SDS	sodiumdodecylsulfate
se	sense

SEM	standard error of the mean
tab	table
Taq	Thermus aquaticus
TCR	T cell receptor
TdT	terminal deoxynucleotidyl transferase
TEMED	N,N,N´,N´-tetramethylethylenediamine
TGFß	transforming growth factor beta
TIL	tumor infiltrating lymphocytes
Treg	regulatory T cell
TßRII	TGFß receptor II
TUNEL	TdT-mediated dUTP-biotin nick end labeling
V	Volt
w/v	weight per volume

2 SUMMARY

Antiestrogens (AE) like tamoxifen belong to the most commonly used drugs in the therapy of estrogen receptor positive (ER+) breast cancer. Nevertheless, relapses frequently occur during treatment indicating development of drug resistance. Concerning the underlying mechanisms, the finding of AE induced TGFß in breast cancer cells appears to be relevant both with respect to TGFß's cell autonomous function as a mediator of cancer progression and its function as an immune regulator. To investigate the potential role of tumor derived, AE induced TGFß as a suppressor of the host's immune response, different *in vitro* assays have been established in this work.

First, a coculture system comprising the hormone sensitive, human breast cancer cell line MCF-7 and primary lymphocytes from healthy female donors was developed. Treatment of MCF-7 cells with either 4-hydroxytamoxifen (OHT), an active metabolite of the prodrug tamoxifen, or fulvestrant/ICI 182.780 (ICI) caused mRNA downregulation of effector molecules like perforin (PRF1), granzyme B (GzmB) and Fas ligand (FasL) in activated cytotoxic CD8+ T cells. These results were confirmed by western blot analysis. The same coculture system revealed an increase in Foxp3 mRNA expression in naïve CD4+ T cells, when MCF-7 cells were treated with OHT or ICI. To exclude transient, activation induced expression of Foxp3 mRNA without development of regulatory T cells (Treg), CD4+ T lymphocytes from MCF-7 cell cocultures were assessed in a suppressor assay with freshly isolated autologous T helper cells. Activation induced proliferation was significantly reduced by T cells from AE treated cocultures as seen by BrdU incorporation. All effects were reversible with a TGFß neutralizing antibody. Moreover, a direct impact of AE on the expression of the investigated lymphocyte molecules could be excluded. To assess the implications of these results on lymphocyte function, heterologous mixed lymphocyte tumor reactions (MLTR) with MCF-7 cells and peripheral blood mononuclear cells (PBMC) or subpopulations were performed. Application of AE strongly reduced the cytotoxicity of immune cells in a TGFß dependent manner, as suggested by a reversal of this effect using a neutralizing antibody.

Finally, an autologous MLTR was established. To this end, tissue from primary mammary carcinomas was processed into standardized slices or was used to isolate epithelial cell adhesion molecule positive (EpCAM+) tumor cells, which were taken into culture. Tumor infiltrating lymphocytes (TIL) were isolated from the same sample for reactivation with interleukin-2 and subsequent application as effector cells. The AE treatment of tumor cells and slices gave rise to enhanced Foxp3 expression of TIL/PBMC and decreased the number of apoptotic tumor cells as

11

seen in a TUNEL assay. A TGFß neutralizing antibody reversed these effects. The work at hand thus provides evidence for an AE treatment induced, TGFß driven immunosuppression in the tumor microenvironment, a mechanism that could critically contribute to development of AE resistance during therapy.

2.1 Zusammenfassung

Antiestrogene (AE) wie Tamoxifen haben sich seit vielen Jahren in der Behandlung des Estrogen-Rezeptor positiven (ER+) Mammakarzinoms bewährt. Allerdings legen häufig auftretende Rückfälle während längerer Einnahme das Entstehen von Resistenzen gegen die Therapie nahe. Die Entdeckung, dass AE den Wachstumsfaktor TGFß in Brustkrebszellen induzieren, hat sich bei der Aufklärung der zugrunde liegenden Mechanismen solcher Resistenzen als sehr hilfreich erwiesen. Neben direkten, sowohl tumorfördernden, als auch tumorhemmenden Effekten auf maligne Zellen, kann TGFß auch eine wichtige Rolle in der Modulation und Suppression der gegen den Tumor gerichteten Immunantwort innehaben. Um letzteres im Rahmen der AE-Wirkung zu untersuchen, wurden in der vorliegenden Arbeit verschiedene Zellkultur-Versuche durchgeführt. Zunächst wurde ein Kokultursystem entwickelt, um die Wirkung von AE-behandelten Tumorzellen auf die Expression von Effektormolekülen in Lymphozyten zu analysieren. Die Behandlung der hormonsensitiven Brustkrebs Zelllinie MCF-7 mit den AE 4-Hydroxy-Tamoxifen (OHT) oder Fulvestrant/ICI 182.780 (ICI) führte zu einer Herabregulierung zytotoxischer Effektormoleküle, wie Perforin, Granzym B und dem Fas Liganden in kokultivierten CD8+ T-Zellen. Dieser Effekt wurde sowohl für die mRNA, als auch die entsprechenden Proteine gezeigt. Analog wurde eine erhöhte Transkription des für die Differenzierung regulatorischer T-Zellen (Treg) verantwortlichen Transkriptionsfaktors Foxp3 in CD4+ T-Zellen nach AE-Behandlung der MCF-7 Zellen nachgewiesen. Die resultierende T-Zell-Population verminderte die Proliferation aktivierter autologer CD4+ T-Zellen, was anhand von BrdU-Einbau in neusynthetisierte DNA gemessen wurde. Bei der Aufklärung dieser Effekte konnte der direkte Einfluss durch AE auf die Lymphozyten zu Gunsten einer TGFß-abhängigen Regulierung ausgeschlossen werden. Um die Wirkung von AE-induziertem TGFß in den MCF-7 Zellen auf die Funktion von Immunzellen aufzudecken, wurde ein heterologer zellbasierter Zytotoxizitätstest (mixed lymphocyte tumor reaction, MLTR) durchgeführt. Die Fähigkeit MCF-7 Zielzellen abzutöten war sowohl in der Gesamtpopulation peripherer, mononukleärer Blutzellen (PBMC), als auch in isolierten CD8+ T-Lymphozyten oder natürlicher Killer (NK) Zellen stark herabgesetzt, wenn die Tumorzellen mit AE behandelt wurden. Die Zugabe eines TGFß neutralisierenden Antikörpers führte zur Aufhebung dieses Effekts. Für eine autologe MLTR wurden aus primären Mammakarzinomen genormte Gewebsschnitte hergestellt und in Kultur genommen. Zugleich wurden sowohl Tumorzellen mittels des spezifischen Oberflächenmarkers EpCAM (epitheliales Zelladhäsionsmolekül), als auch Tumor-infiltrierende Lymphozyten (TIL) aus der gleichen Probe isoliert. Letztere kamen als Effektorzellen zum

Einsatz, nachdem sie mit Interleukin-2 stimuliert, bzw. reaktiviert wurden. Während der autologen MLTR mit Tumorschnitten oder –zellen kam es unter AE-Behandlung zu einem Anstieg der Foxp3 mRNA in TIL, was eine erhöhte Entstehungsrate von immunsuppressiven Treg-Zellen nahelegt. Diese Hypothese untermauernd konnte in einer anschließenden TUNEL-Färbung der Nachweis erbracht werden, dass in den AE-behandelten MLTR-Ansätzen weniger Tumorzellen durch Apoptose abgetötet werden. Auch hier wurde die Umkehrbarkeit durch einen neutralisierenden TGFß Antikörper demonstriert.

Die Ergebnisse dieser Arbeit sprechen für die These, dass die Therapie mit AE zu einer TGFß-vermittelten Unterdrückung des Immunsystems in der unmittelbaren Umgebung des Tumors führen kann. Der hieraus resultierende Überlebensvorteil für den Tumor kann wesentlich zur Entstehung einer AE-Resistenz während der Behandlung beitragen.

3 Introduction

3.1 Breast cancer

Mammary carcinomas represent the most common form of cancer in females living in western countries. In Germany it accounts for 28% of all cancers diagnosed in women with an incidence of about 57,000 per year (Robert Koch-Institut, 2008). The occurrence in men is rather seldom and constitutes a fraction of less than 1% of all reported cases. One has to differentiate between sporadic forms, which arise from DNA damage and somatic mutations in breast cells during a lifetime and hereditary burden leading to so called familial breast cancer. Mutations in dominant susceptibility genes like BRCA1 or BRCA2 are inheritable and appear to be responsible for about 5% of all breast cancer cases (Emery, 2001). Therefore, the bulk of the disease has to be traced back to acquired forms. The discussion concerning underlying risk factors comprises e.g. nulliparity or late pregnancy (30 years and older), use of oral contraceptives and post-menopausal hormone therapy, early menarche, late menopause and others (American cancer society). Strikingly, most of these criteria are related to an increased lifetime exposure to steroidal sex hormones like estrogens. Target tissues for their mitogenic actions can be found in reproductive organs like the breast, e.g. epithelial cells in the mammary glands and the adjacent milk ducts. These tissues constitute hormone responsive sites, which are at the same time the potential origin for arising carcinomas. Thus, the high abundance of estrogen receptor expression in breast cancer – about 70% of all mammary carcinomas are ER+ (Harvey, 1999) - is a clear result of this interrelation. Receptor activation is caused by binding of 17ß-estradiol and positively regulates growth and development of both healthy and malignant tissue e.g. via induction of growth factors (Osborne, 1990). Due to this tumor promoting action, the estrogen receptor is an important target for the therapy of breast cancer.

3.2 Estrogen receptors and antiestrogens

The estrogen receptor belongs to the nuclear receptor superfamily of ligand-regulated transcription factors. To date, two subtypes called ERα and ERß have been identified. Binding of their natural ligands causes receptor dimerization and translocation into the nucleus (Rachez C, 2001) where N- and C-terminal activation functions (AF-1 and AF-2) lead to transcription of

15

target genes (Nilsson S., 2001). The receptor complex can either bind to estrogen response elements (ERE) in target gene promotor regions (Klinge, 2001) or to serum response elements (SRE) through protein-protein interaction with other transcription factors like activating protein 1 (Ap1). The estrogen receptor does not only exhibit affintiy for endogenous/physiological ligands like estradiol, but also for a panel of other substances, each of which induces a specific conformation of the receptor protein. This spatial arrangement entails binding of different either activating or inhibiting cofactors, which are necessary for transcriptional activity (Shang, 2000). Because the ratio of these coactivators and corepressors can vary between different tissues, a ligand can be an agonist in one cell type, while acting antagonistically in another. To modulate the estrogen receptor response, especially in the treatment of hormone responsive breast cancer, molecules referred to as selective estrogen receptor modulators (SERM) or pure antiestrogens have been designed. Based on their chemical structures, they can be divided into three categories: triphenylethylenes like tamoxifen, nonsteroidal compounds like raloxifen and steroidal compounds, e.g. fulvestrant.

Tamoxifen and tamoxifen metabolites like endoxifen or 4-hydroxytamoxifen in particular compete with estrogens for binding to the estrogen receptor. Tamoxifen induces a receptor conformation, which blocks AF-2 function but leaves AF-1 in an active state. As a consequence of this just fractional inhibition, it is termed a partial antiestrogen (McDonnell, 1995). In this context, tamoxifen is a drug with the above described tissue-depending action profile, causing antagonistic effects in hormone responsive breast cancer but acts as an agonist in bone tissue.

Fulvestrant (ICI 182.780) on the other hand is able to stall both activation functions of the estrogen receptor, thereby leading to a complete inhibition of its transcriptional activity. As opposed to tamoxifen no agonistic effects have been discovered. Due to this feature fulvestrant is classified as a pure antiestrogen (McDonnell, 1995).

3.3 Antiestrogen resistance

The endocrine therapy of breast cancer, especially the application of tamoxifen is considered as an effective approach, which includes several benefits. Besides the pivotal criterion that adjuvant treatment with tamoxifen decreases the recurrency rate to about 50% and reduces the number of breast cancer deaths by one-third (EBCTCG, 2005), osteoporosis preventing effects were also shown. Additionally, tamoxifen causes a decrease in cardiovascular disease (Jordan, 1993). Nevertheless, one-third of patients who received 5 years of tamoxifen treatment developed recurrencies during a 15 years follow-up time (EBCTCG, 2005). Second line therapy with pure antiestrogens like fulvestrant seems to overcome tamoxifen related resistance. However, well-founded clinical trials concerning their longterm efficiency are still missing. In general, second line therapeutics could also be susceptible to similar resistance mechanisms as seen in course of tamoxifen treatment.

Resistance to antiestrogen therapy can emerge from either intrinsic (*de novo*) or acquired mechanisms in tumor cells. Lack of estrogen receptor expression is considered as an *a priori* and cell inherent feature leading to no or weak response, whereas some estrogen receptor negative tumors show antiestrogen sensitivity. Another intrinsic mechanism lies in the different genetic variants of the polymorphic enzyme cytochrome P450 (CYP) 2D6, which is necessesary for conversion of the prodrug tamoxifen into its active metabolites (e.g. endoxifen, 4-hydroxytamoxifen). CYP 2D6 variants with a poor metabolizing phenotype can be found in about 8% of Caucasian women and are associated with poor clinical outcome (Schroth, 2009).

Antiestrogen treatment can result in a selection of estrogen independent cells from heterologous tumor cell populations. As a consequence, most of the acquired mechanisms in drug resistant breast cancers emerge from changes and deregulation in estrogen signaling networks. This can directly concern the expression of the estrogen receptor, the loss of which was seen in about 15-20% of biopsies from tamoxifen resistant breast tumors in a study by Gutierrez *et al.* (2005). In contrast, ER mutations occurred rather seldom (<1%) (Roodi, 1995). Another important way to overcome antiestrogen induced growth inhibition is the ligand-independent activation of the estrogen receptor through phosphorylation. Among the prerequisites for this bypass of estrogenic action is the cross-talk with other mitogenic pathways, often correlated with overexpression of growth factor receptors like EGFR, IGFR or Her2 (Arpino, 2008).

Besides, antiestrogenic effects on the signaling of the estrogen receptor include regulation of growth factor expression and secretion. The resulting expression and activation pattern is shifted from a mitogenic towards a growth inhibitory profile with a significant increase in TGFß levels. TGFß is known to repress tumorigenesis and to act as a suppressor in early stage malignancies. As opposed to TGFß2, the transcription of TGFß1 is not enhanced but more active TGFß1 protein can be detected in the supernatants of the breast cancer cell line MCF-7 after antiestrogen application (Knabbe, 1987). In correlation to these findings there is enhanced TGFß2 mRNA expression in biopsies of tamoxifen responding breast cancer during treatment (MacCallum, 1996). Furthermore, serum levels of TGFß2 in tamoxifen responding patients are elevated during the first 4-8 weeks of treatment (Kopp, 1995). But aside from TGFßs tumor suppressive role in the beginning, its longterm effects are more complex, as demonstrated by a frequent switch to

17

promoting effects in late stage tumors. The underlying deregulation of TGFß signaling can play an important role in antiestrogen resistance (Lippmann 1988; Knabbe, 1996; Arteaga, 1999).

3.4 TGFß

The growth factor TGFß is a 25 kDa homodimeric protein with a highly pleiotropic action profile. Depending on the target cell type, its differentiation status and additional stimuli, TGFß can induce proliferation, apoptosis, regulate differentiation, migration and adhesion (Sporn, 1988). Moreover, it is also involved in the formation of extracellular matrix.

Like bone morphogenetic proteins (BMP), activins and inhibins it belongs to the TGFß superfamily. To date, 3 highly homologous isoforms called TGFß1, 2 and 3 have been discovered in humans with TGFß1 being the predominant form expressed in the immune system (Li, 2006). All isoforms are expressed and secreted as precursor molecules, which are not able to bind to and activate the TGFß receptor complex. The biologically inactive form is composed of the latency associated protein (LAP), the latent TGFß binding protein (LTBP) and the actual bioactive TGFß molecule. The resulting retention of active TGFß in the latency complex constitutes an additional level of regulation because the effector protein deposited in such way can be activated as and when required (Annes, 2003). A variety of molecules and mechanisms for activation of latent TGFß have been described ranging from proteolytical cleavage by matrix metalloproteinases (Yu, 2000) and interaction with integrins to activation by reactive oxygen species (Barcellos-Hoff, 1994), low pH or shear-forces (Lyons, 1988; Ahamed J, 2008).

The bioactive form binds to a heteromeric transmembrane receptor serine/threonine kinase complex, which in turn is activated. This leads to either canonical Smad protein based TGFß signaling or to activation of MAP kinase pathways.

3.5 The dual role of TGFß in carcinogenesis

3.5.1 TGFß as a tumor suppressor

During tumorigenesis TGFß appears to play an intricate either suppressive or promoting role, which might seem contradictory at first glance. Experiments performed with human mammary epithelial cells (Valverius, 1989) and transgenic mouse models suggest that TGFß is involved in growth control and homeostasis of epithelial tissues. In this context, TGFß has been shown to downregulate the proliferation driving transcription factor c-myc, thereby inducing a de-repression of the cyclin-dependent kinase inhibitors p15Ink4b and p21Cip1. Besides its ability to inhibit cell proliferation and to maintain tissue architecture, it can influence DNA damage response, thus preventing genomic instability and inducing apoptosis (Engle, 1999; Glick, 1996; Yang, 2002). However, the mechanistical background of cell death induction in epithelial cells is still not well-understood and seems to be context-dependent.

Tissue specific TGFß overexpression by means of a mammary gland-selective mouse mammary tumor virus (MMTV) promotor caused a delay in mammary gland development and inhibited carcinogen-induced tumor formation in the breast (Pierce, 1995). Furthermore, both MMTV promotor/enhancer driven expression of a dominant negative TGFß receptor II (TßRII) and TßRII-antisense RNA led to mammary epithelial hyperplasia. There are conflicting data concerning the spontaneous formation of mammary carcinoma when targeting TßRII or Smad proteins in transgenic mice models (Gorska, 2003; Forrester, 2005). But several studies revealed that treating these animals with 7,12-dimethyl-benz[α] anthracene (MDBA) or crossbreeding them with MMTV-polyomavirus middle T antigen (PyVmT) or MMTV-TGFα transgenic mice resulted in a strong increase in tumor formation. Thus, TGFß signaling inhibition by silencing TßRII or Smad proteins does not seem to drive neoplasia itself but greatly increases tumor incidence when additional carcinogenic (PyVmT) or mitogenic stimuli (TGFα) are present. The finding that expression of TßRII was detectable in all low-grade human breast cancer but only in 31% of high-grade tumors with high invasive potential seems to confirm the tumor suppressing role of TGFß in humans (Gobbi, 2000).

3.5.2 TGFß as a tumor promoter – autocrine effects

Opposing to the picture of TGFß action as described above, there is a plethora of publications in which TGFß (over-) expression in tumors is shown to correlate with a more aggressive phenotype and a poor prognosis (Derynck, 2001; Gold, 1999). To elucidate the underlying mechanisms of this outcome, a large number of *in vitro* studies were performed to supplement and deepen the clinical evidence. It is getting clear that during growth and adaption to their environment, tumor cells become insensitive to the growth inhibitory effects of TGFß. This switch in response includes changes in TGFß cell autonomous functions and a stronger accentuation of its paracrine effects, many of which are considered as benefical for tumor development and metastasis.

Alterations in autocrine effects of TGFß seldomly comprise complete loss of signaling. Rather, an imbalance concerning the activation of different TGFß signal pathways comes into force, emphasizing tumor promoting PI3K and various MAPK cascades at the expense of tumor suppressive Smad signaling. This change can result from mutations or epigenetic mechanisms, which decrease TßRII expression (Kim, 2000). Another obvious way to bypass the Smad pathway is diminution or loss of Smad protein expression or activation as seen in a study by Xie *et al.* (2002), where absence of Smad 4 or phosphorylated Smad 2 was shown to correlate with a poor outcome. Interestingly, partial retention of Smad signaling favours changes in cell morphology and function, which are linked to invasivness, whereas its complete absence leads to reduced migratory potential and metastasis (Massagué, 2008).

Furthermore, there is an increasing body of evidence that cross-talk with mitogenic pathways can convert tumor suppressive TGFß signaling into a stimulus, which facilitates migration and tissue invasion. Again, the Smad pathway is impaired for the benefit of alternative signal cascades, as exemplified by epidermal growth factor signaling induced stabilization of the Smad corepressor homeodomain protein TG-interacting factor (TGIF) (Lo, 2001). Another interface for conversion of suppressive TGFß pathways into pro-migratory and –invasive stimuli is the cross-talk with overxpressed Her2/neu signaling (Seton-Rogers, 2004). The latter finding is of high significance as about 30% of human mammary carcinoma exhibit increased Her2/neu expression (Slamon, 1987). Of central importance for tumor migration and invasion processes is a loss of cell-cell adhesion, often accompanied by conversion of malignant epithelial cells into a fibroblastic phenotype (Huber, 2005). This change in cell morphology and function is referred to as epithelial- mesenchymal transduction (EMT), an event, which also plays a desicive role during embryonic development. TGFß is an important regulator in physiological as well as in pathophysiological EMT (Xu, 2009). The tumor suppressor and cell adhesion molecule E-cadherin is often downregulated in tumors and its overexpression can prevent invasive behaviour. The TGFß induced transcription factors Snail and Slug can inhibit E-cadherin expression (Siegel, 2003), thereby allowing malignant cells for dissociation from united cell structure.

New insights in the switch of tumor response to TGFß were also derived from investigations concerning epigenetic regulation. In gastric cancer enhanced expression of the micro-RNA cluster miR-106b-25 led to abolition of TGFß induced cell cycle arrest and apoptosis by inhibiting the cyclin-dependent kinase inhibitor p21CIP1 and BIM, a proapoptotic mediator (Petrocca, 2008).

3.5.3 TGFß as a tumor promoter – paracrine effects

Beyond changes in receptor signaling, paracrine effects of TGFß also play an important role in tumorigenesis. Latent TGFß is sequestered in the extracellular matrix where its activation can render the microenvironment tumor-promoting, e.g. through induction of angiogenesis (Roberts, 1986; Gajdusek, 1993). The formation of tumor interfusing blood vessels leads to enhanced supply of oxygen and nutrients, which are critical for growth. Moreover, access to the blood system facilitates dissemination and subsequent formation of metastasis. The required generation of a local pro-angiogenic environment can be induced by effects of TGFß signaling and a hypoxic milieu, the synergy of which lead to an increase in vascular endothelial growth factor (VEGF) mRNA expression (Sanchez-Elsner, 2001). Another central mediator of angiogenesis, the connective tissue growth factor (CTGF), can also directly be targeted by TGFß signaling. In human breast cancer a high TGFß mRNA expression correlated with increased microvessel density (de Jong, 1998).

In addition, paracrine effects of TGFß are known to orchestrate processes of invasion and metastasis. Tobin *et al.* (2002) overexpressed TGFß1 in TGFß responsive MDA-231 cells, thereby slowing down their *in vitro* proliferation. However, after inoculation in mice these cells showed accelerated growth and a pronounced metastatic phenotype. Exclusion of autocrine effects by cotransfection with a dominant negative TßRII reduced *in vivo* growth rates but did not affect incidence of lung metastasis. This is pointing to the crucial role of paracrine TGFß signaling in invasion and formation of metastasis. It has been shown in our group that an insertion polymorphism in the TGFß2 promotor causes enhanced promoter activity. The resulting increase in TGFß2 protein, which was seen on tumor sections from breast cancer patients, correlated with enhanced lymph node metastasis (Beisner, 2006). Consistent with these results, there are several studies showing correlation of high TGFß levels with a more aggressive and invasive tumor phenotype (Friedman, 1995; Maehara, 1999; Padua, 2009). Among the responsible mechanisms could be TGFß controlled expression and activation of matrix metalloproteinases, which are involved in the degradation of extracellular matrix (ECM).

Of further importance with respect to ECM degradation could be chemotactic recruitment and modulation of macrophages through TGFß (Condeelis, 2006; Byrne, 2008). Generally, paracrine action of TGFß plays a central role in the modulation of cells from both the innate and the adaptive branch of the immune system. In addition, TGFß is among the chief mediators of tumor evasion from immune surveillance.

3.6 Role of TGFß in tumor immunology

The evolution of inherent systems to protect organisms from infections already started in bacteria. Beginning with the expression of restriction enzymes to repel bacteriophage viruses, this process led to the development of sophisticated defense mechanisms in vertebrates comprising both specialized cell types and molecules. The simpliest definition of their function is the ability to tell apart foreign and self structures. This includes the antigen-mediated recognition of malignant cells as a target for eradication. Typical tumor antigens can be derived from oncogenic viruses, mutated or overexpressed (oncogenic) proteins and proteins, which are normally expressed during embryogenesis but actually disappear in the fully developed organism. Yet, despite the presence of cancer associated antigens and immune cells specific for them, tumors obviously manage to overcome the resulting antitumor immune response. One pivotal mechanism for tumor escape from immune surveillance is the local expression of immunosuppressive molecules like TGFß (Wrzesinski, 2007). Its suppressive role is established for both branches of the immune system, the innate and the adaptive one (Li, 2006).

3.6.1 Effects on the adaptive immune response

The adaptive immune system is composed of T and B lymphocytes expressing highly specific antigen receptors, which exhibit a vast diversity due to somatic hypermutation and intense recombination activity in the encoding genes. They originate from hematopoietic stem cells in the bone marrow and undergo maturation, during which they are subject to selection processes eradicating those cells with affinity to antigens naturally produced in the body. Matured lymphocytes are released from the bone marrow (B cells) or the thymus (T cells) into the periphery where they circulate in an inactive status. High affinity binding of the T or B cell receptors to the appropriate antigen is necessary for activation and differentiation into an effector cell.

TGFß is known to be a master regulator of differentiation, homeostasis, proliferation and effector function of both T and B cells (Li, 2006; Li, 2008). Its crucial role in maintaining well-balanced immune functions is illustrated by the phenotype of TGFß knockout mice, which suffer from severe autoimmune defects. This includes massive lymphocyte infiltration of lymphatic and non-lymphatic organs, hyperproliferation and spontaneous differentiation into and activation of effector cells, accompanied by inflammation processes (Shull, 1992). T cell specific expression of a dominant negative TßRII in mice led to a highly similar phenotype (Gorelik, 2000).

Accordingly, TGFß is considered to be a negative regulator of T cells, keeping their proliferation and activation in check. Concerning its ambiguous role in immunopathology, TGFß is not only involved in preventing potential autoimmune reactions by repression of overshooting T lymphocyte activity. Furthermore, it is frequently (over-) expressed in cancer and, as T lymphocytes are among the key effector cells in the prevention and eradication of cancer, can act as a suppressor of antitumor immune responses.

The affected T cells constitute a heterogeneous population consisting of different subsets with distinct functions. Basically, they are divided into CD8+ T cells with cytolytic properties and CD4+ helper T cells, which exhibit a higher phenotypic plasticity. Based on the cytokine composition and other stimuli during CD4+ T cell activation, they can differentiate into specialized subsets in order to orchestrate the emerging immune response. The former paradigm proposed a dual differentiation model either generating a Th1 response, which stimulates the cellular immunity, or a Th2 response. The latter is focussed on the humoral immune system and mainly induces B cell proliferation and antibody production. This dual model has recently been extended by the discovery of another distinct T helper cell subset, which is characterized by expression of interleukin 17 and is therefore referred to as the Th17 subpopulation (Harrington, 2005). Another subset with a better established role in antitumor immune responses and a pivotal function for the entire immune system is provided by immunosuppressive regulatory T cells (T reg). TGFß is an influential regulator of all mentioned T cell subpopulations.

3.6.2 Cytotoxic CD8+ T cells

Cytotoxic CD8+ T lymphocytes (CTL) are critical for lysis of tumor cells during an antitumor response (Baxevanis, 1994). After activation by dendritic cells (DC) or macrophages, which can present tumor associated antigens (TAA) and stimulate lymphocytes, CTL are able to directly kill malignant cells after recognition via antigen specific T cell receptors (TCR). Normally, stimulation of the TCR by binding the appropriate antigen presented on major histocompatibility complex I (MHCI) launches target cell lysis programs in activated CTL. This comprises activation of the granule exocytosis pathway and Fas ligand (FasL) mediated induction of apoptosis. The former is based on the release of cytolytic effector molecules deposited in vesicles, which are fused to the lymphocyte´s cell membrane after target cell recognition. Discharge of the pore forming protein perforin and caspase activating enzymes referred to as granzymes have been proven to trigger apoptosis in attacked cells (Barry, 2002). Furthermore,

23

CTL exert their effector function by secreting proinflammatory cytokines like interferon γ (IFNγ).

Whereas TGFß seems to promote thymic CD8+ T cell differentiation in mice (Li, 2008) its effects on peripheral CTL are mainly detrimental. Among the mechanistical aspects of its suppressive impact on CTL is the Smad 3 mediated inhibition of interleukin 2 (IL-2) promotor activity, TGFß signaling induced upregulation of cyclin dependent kinase inhibitors p15 and p21 and decrease in cell cycle driving factors like c-myc and cyclin D2 (Ma, 2006; Kehrl, 1986). Both TGFß caused reduction of the T cell activating lymphokine IL-2 and cell cycle-mediators like cyclins result in proliferation inhibition. Moreover, TGFß blocks the differentiation from naïve CD8+ T cell into fully activated CTL, basically by inhibiting the expression of effector molecules like perforin, granzymes and FasL (Smyth, 1991; Thomas, 2005). These impairments in CTL proliferation and function appear to be essential for the TGFß driven escape from elimination by the immune system, which is frequently seized by tumors. This is exemplified by T cell specific blockade of TGFß signaling, which leads to eradication of malignant cells in tumor bearing mice (Gorelik and Flavell, 2001). Similar evidence derives from application of TGFß neutralizing antibodies. Moreover, in a study by Thomas and (Thomas, 2005) EL4 thymoma cells, known to express TGFß, and EL4 cells transfected with a short hairpin RNAi targeting TGFß were injected in mice. The resulting decrease of TGFß expression in transfected EL4 cells caused a delay of tumor development. The expression of a soluble TßRII in EL4 cells turned out to be even more benefical for the survival of inoculated mice, as only 20% died in comparison to 75% (TGFß-RNAi EL4 cells) and 80% (WT EL4 cells) lethality, respectively. Furthermore, tumor-specific CTL were isolated from inoculated mice and assessed for effector molecule expression. Neutralization of TGFß led to restored perforin and granzyme protein levels.

Yet, TGFßs suppressive effects on CTL are not axiomatic but rather context-dependent. For instance, already activated CD8+ T lymphocytes are hardly suppressed by TGFß. Furthermore, addition of exogenous IL-2 to TGFß inhibited CTL can partially reactivate their ability to proliferate and both 4-1BBL, a T cell costimulatory molecule expressed on antigen presenting cells (APC), and interleukin-12 are able to restore TGFß inhibited differentiation (Kim, 2005).

3.6.3 Regulatory T cells

The existence of immune cells with suppressive potential has been proposed more than 3 decades ago (Gershon, 1975) but the according investigations stagnated for several years. The more recent discovery of a CD4+CD25+ (interleukin receptor α chain) T cell subpopulation, characterized by expression of the transcription factor Foxp3 and its ability to suppress other immune cells, has considerably revitalized this research field. A central role of Foxp3 expressing regulatory T cells (Treg) in immune homeostasis and peripheral tolerance is stressed by studies with Foxp3 knockout mice, which display a phenotype similar to that seen in TGFß knockout mice, including a fatal lymphoproliferative disease (Lyon, 1990). The converse approach, Foxp3 overexpression in mice resulted in massively depressed immune functions (Khattri, 2001). Relating to humans, dysfunctional Foxp3 caused by a rare mutation leads to an autoimmune disease referred to as IPEX (immunodysregulation polyendocrinopathy enteropathy X-linked syndrome). Besides expression of Foxp3 and CD25, Treg can be characterized by surface molecules like CTLA-4 (cytotoxic T lymphocyte activation-4) and GITR (glucocorticoid induced tumor necrosis factor receptor).

In general, regulatory characteristics are not restricted to a unique cell type. Aside from CD8+CD28- T cells, CD4-CD8- T cells and natural killer T (NKT) cells all showing suppressive potential (Shevach, 2006), the CD4+ Treg population can be divided into 2 basic categories. Naturally occuring CD4+CD25+ Treg (nTreg), which develop in the thymus during T cell maturation and Treg, which are induced from naïve CD4+ T cells in the periphery (iTreg). The latter can be subclassified into Tr1 and Th3 regulatory cells abundantly found in the intestine or generated in oral tolerance, respectively. In all cases, TGFß holds an important, yet controversially discussed function in differentiation and suppressive activity. Conflicting data concerning the role of TGFß in the development of nTreg comes from studies using T cell specific expression of dominant negative forms of TßRII in mice (Schramm, 2003; Gorelik, 2000). However, a more recent report corroborates the concept that loss of TGFß signaling in CD4+ T cells does not affect normal development of nTreg in the thymus but significantly reduced their maintenance in the periphery (Li, 2006). Furthermore, the *in vitro* generation of iTreg from naïve human CD4+CD25- T cells was achieved by application of TGFß, which resulted in upregulation of Foxp3 and development of suppressive properties (Fantini, 2004). *In vivo* studies in mice confirmed the crucial role of TGFß in peripheral iTreg induction by transient transgenic expression of TGFß in pancreatic islets of diabetic mice. This approach led to the site specific generation of CD4+CD25+Foxp3+ iTreg and protection against autoimmune reactions (Peng, 2004).

Both Treg inducibility by TGFß and frequent TGFß expression in cancer suggests an involvement of Treg in tumor immunology. In deed, increased levels of Foxp3+ Treg were seen in peripheral blood of tumor patients (Ormandy, 2005). With regard to their suppressive role,

25

Treg can undermine antitumor immune responses, which should normally be elicited in the case of recognition by tumor specific lymphocytes. This was illustrated by a study from Shimizu *et al.* (1999), were removal of Treg in tumor bearing mice caused an increased antitumor immunity. Accordingly, enhanced generation of Treg via immunization with self antigens in mice led to accelerated development of 3-methylcholanthrene (MCA)-induced tumors, which was again inhibited by depletion of CD4+ or CD25+ T cells (Nishikawa, 2005). Moreover, abundancy of Foxp3+ lymphocytes in tumor tissue of breast cancer patients was correlated with a poor prognosis concerning late-relapse and reduced overall survival (Bates, 2006). Thus, regarding their funtion in preventing autoimmunity on the one hand and their role in tumorigenesis on the other, Treg can feature both beneficial and deleterious effects for the organism.

Due to the common acknowledgment of their importance and intense investigations, there is significant progress relating to the detailed mechanisms, by which Treg suppress other immune cells. Cell-cell contact dependent and independent inhibition of effector T cells through membrane bound or soluble immunesuppressive factors like TGFß or interleukin-10 has been described (Shevach, 2006). Another contact-independent mechanism was deduced from high expression of the interleukin-2 receptor α chain (CD25). This feature could lead to a competitive binding of the mitogen IL-2, thereby causing failed conversion of naïve into effector T cells and at the same time further expansion of the Treg compartment (Thornton, 1998). A more drastic Treg mechanism lies in granzyme and perforin mediated cytolysis of NK cells and CTL, which was seen in Treg induced suppression of tumor clearance (Cao, 2007). Beyond direct effects on effector T cell function, Treg can also impair T cell activation through modulation of antigen presenting cells (APC). APC belong to innate immune system and are indispensable in the initiation of adaptive immune responses, e.g. due to the expression of T cell costimulatory molecules like CD80 or CD86. These proteins were shown to be downregulated by Treg (Cederbom, 2000).

3.6.4 T helper cells

During activation and acquisition of effector functions, T helper cell differentiation can be skewed towards varying phenotypes according to incoming T cell receptor (TCR) and costimulatory signals in addition to the present cytokine composition (O´Garra, 1998). This plasticity makes sure that the emerging immune response is adequate for the present pathogenic target. Intracellular infections and malignant transformation require a cell directed immune

26

response, mainly leading to induction of CTL and enhanced macrophage activity. In contrast to this so called Th1 response, extracellular pathogens and parasites usually provoke a Th2 response, in the course of which B cell production of antibodies and stimulation of mast cells and eosinophils is initiated. Both differentiation types incluce the expression of a specific cytokine pattern, whereas Th1 cytokines (IL-2, IL-12, IFNγ, TNFα, etc.) inhibit the development Th2 responses (IL-4, -5, -6, -10, -13, etc.) and the other way around. As described above, an additional T helper cell phenotpye referred to as Th17 has recently been discovered. The characteristic Th17 cytokines include IL-17 and IL-22. Similar to the expression of Foxp3 in Treg, there is a lineage specific induction of transcription factors for the known T helper cell subsets, comprising T-bet (T-box transcription factor TBX21) for Th1 cells, GATA-3 (GATA binding factor 3) for Th2 cells and RORγt (retinoid-related orphan receptor-gamma) for Th17 lymphocytes.

Mice with T cell specific expression of a dominant negative TβRII showed spontaneous differentiation of Th1 or Th2 cells (Gorelik, 2000). Accordingly, TGFβ application downregulated T-bet and GATA-3 protein levels via decreased TCR-induced activation of the Tec kinase Itk, less Ca2+ influx and thereby reduced NFAT (nuclear factor of activated T cells) activation (Chen, 2003). The direct inhibition of IL-2 and the Th1 associated factors IFNγ and TNFα (tumor necrosis factor α) further emphasizes the repressive role of TGFβ in T cell activation and differentiation. However, Th17 cell differentiation – at least *in vitro* - seems to constitute an exception, as it requires TGFβ in addition to interleukin-6. Interestingly, TGFβ induction of either Th17 cells or Treg appears to be mutually exclusive, which renders their induction as competitive events. Th17 cells appear to be involved in autoimmunity and inflammation, whereas their role in tumor immunology has to be further investigated. Ambigous data exist regarding Th1 and Th2 cells in the antitumor response but there are studies showing increased systemic Th2 cytokine levels in cancer patients with advanced tumors (Wittke, 1999). Investigations of Kumar *et al.* (2006) uncovered an imbalance in IL-12 (Th1) and IL-10 (Th2) serum levels for the benefit of a Th2 response in brain tumor patients. The predominance of a Th2 differentiation is thought to be utile for tumorigenesis, as it goes hand in hand with the lack of a cell directed Th1 response and includes expression of suppressive molecules like IL-10 (Lucey DR, 1996). Interestingly, differentiated Th1 cells seem to be more susceptible to inhibitory TGFβ effects than Th2 cells, the effector cytokine production of which is not affected by TGFβ (Ludviksson, 2000).

3.6.5 Effects on the innate immune response

Innate immunity is constituted by a more primordial part of the immune system, which arose much earlier in evolution than the adaptive one. Aside from mechanical barriers like the skin and chemical barriers, generated by means of antimicrobial molecules, the innate immune system in vertebrates is composed of different specialized cell types. The most significant difference between innate and adaptive immune cells lies in the specificity of antigen recognition, whereas innate immune cells display a more generic detection of pathogens due to the expression of pattern recognition receptors (PRR). As a consequence, initiation of a robust innate response is much faster because there is no necessity for clonal expansion of a few cells with high specificity for the present antigen. However, in contrary to the adaptive immunity, the generation of long-lasting immunological memory against pathogens is missing.

A crucial role is hold by antigen-presenting cells (APC), which can internalize pathogens or apoptotic vesicles of malignant cells, process them and present the resulting antigen peptides on major histocompatibility complexes (MHC). Together with costimulatory ligands like B7-1 (CD80) and B7-2 (CD86), the MHC associated antigens can activate appropriate specific lymphocytes via their TCR, thereby inducing an adaptive immune response. TGFß inhibits the maturation and function of APC like dendritic cells (DC) and macrophages. Its inclusion during activation of DC downregulates MHCII as well as costimulatory molecules, which leads to failed activation of lymphocytes (Geissmann, 1999). In macrophages, TGFß inhibits both the expression of PRR and activation associated inflammatory mediators like TNFα, macrophage inflammatory protein 1α (MIP-1α) and MIP-2 (Han, 2000; Bogdan, 1992). Furthermore, similar to its effects on DC, antigen presenting functions of macrophages are also impaired by TGFß induced downregulation of MHCII and costimulatory molecules like CD40 (Takeuchi, 1998).

Natural killer cells originate from the same hematopoietic progenitor cell type like lymphocytes but lack expression of specific TCR. As a consequence, they are classified as representatives of the innate immune system. Like CTL, NK cells are critical in the prevention and clearance of tumors, which they can kill without prior activation or immunization. Once more, TGFßs central role in immunity is fortified by a strong regulatory potential on NK cells. Its effects include downregulation of activating immunoreceptor natural killer group 2, member D (NKG2D), reduced IFNγ production and less antitumor reactivity (Kopp, 2009). TGFß-mediated inhibition of NK cells not only originates from secretion by tumor cells but can also be utilized by tumor associated Treg, as reported in a study by (Ghiringhelli, 2006).

Aims of this work

The aim of this study was to elucidate immunological implications of antiestrogen (AE) induced TGFß in mammary carcinoma cells. It can be reasoned that AE mediated increase in TGFß, the immunosuppressive role of which is well-established, could constitute a benefit for cancer cells through a local attenuation of antitumor immune responses. This putative mechanism could critically contribute to frequently occurring resistances during AE treatment.

Both the cytotoxicity of CD8+ T cells (CTL) and the induction of regulatory CD4+ T cells (Treg) are known to be influenced by TGFß. These T cell subsets, which hold central functions in tumor immunology, were monitored for potential effects of AE treated tumor cells on immune responses. Therefore, mRNA and protein expression of cytolytic molecules and specific transcription factors in coculture models as well as effector function in mixed lymphocyte tumor reactions and suppressor assays (for Tregs) was assessed. Both heterologous cytotoxicity tests with the hormone responsive human breast cancer cell line MCF-7 and PBMC from healthy female donors as well as autologous reactions with tissue from breast cancer biopsies and reactivated tumor infiltrating lymphocytes were performed. The influence of antiestrogen treatment on antitumor immune responses was addressed by measuring cell death of tumor cells. Furthermore, the cytokine composition in heterologous mixed lymphocyte tumor reactions and its effect on T helper cell differentiation was analysed.

4 MATERIALS

4.1 Chemicals, reagents and enzymes

100 bp DNA ladder	Gibco BRL, Karlsruhe
2'-deoxyadenosine 5'-triphosphate	Amersham, Braunschweig
2'-deoxycytidine 5'-triphosphate	Amersham, Braunschweig
2'-deoxyguanosine 5'-triphosphate	Amersham, Braunschweig
2'-deoxythymidine 5'-triphosphate	Amersham, Braunschweig
24-well cell culture plates	Nunc, Roskilde, DK
2-mercaptoethanol	Sigma, Deisenhofen
30% acrylamide/bis solution 37.5 : 1	Bio-Rad, München
4-hydroxytamoxifen	Sigma, Deisenhofen
6-well cell culture plates	Nunc, Roskilde, DK
Agarose ultra pure	Gibco BRL, Karlsruhe
Albumine	Sigma, Deisenhofen
Ammoniumperoxidisulfate	Roth, Karlsruhe
Ampicillin	Roth, Karlsruhe
Anti BrdU	Becton Dickinson, USA
Bacto-agar	Becton Dickinson, Erembodegem, Belgium
Biocoll	Biochrom AG, Berlin
Blotting paper	Schleicher & Schüll, Dassel
Bradford reagent	BioRad, München
BrdU	Sigma, Deisenhofen
BSA	Sigma, Deisenhofen
Colistin	Sigma, Deisenhofen
Collagenase	Sigma, Taufkirchen
DMEM	Gibco BRL, Karlsruhe
DMSO	Sigma, Deisenhofen
DNase I	Sigma, Taufkirchen
DTT	Sigma, Deisenhofen
EcoRI	Gibco BRL, Karlsruhe
EDTA	Merck, Darmstadt
EGTA	Merck, Darmstadt

Formaldehyde	Merck, Darmstadt
G418	Sigma, Deisenhofen
Gentamycin	Gibco BRL, Karlsruhe
Glucose	Sigma, Deisenhofen
Glycin	Serva, Heidelberg
HindIII	Gibco BRL, Karlsruhe
ICI 182.780	Tocris, Bristol, UK
Interleukin-2	ImmunoTools, Friesoythe
LB-agar	Sigma, Deisenhofen
LB-medium	Sigma, Deisenhofen
Liforlab®	Oncoscience, Wedel
PMSF	Sigma, Deisenhofen
Ponceau solution	Sigma, Deisenhofen
Potassium chloride	Merck, Darmstadt
Propidium iodide	Sigma, Deisenhofen
Protease	Sigma, Taufkirchen
RNase A	Qiagen, Hilden
SDS	Sigma, Deisenhofen
Sodium chlorid	Merck, Darmstadt
Sodium pyruvate	Gibco BRL, Karlsruhe
Sulfatase	Sigma, Deisenhofen
SuperSignal® West Dura Extended Duration Substrate	Thermo Fisher Scientififc, Ulm
T75 cell culture flasks	Corning, Wiesbaden
Taq-DNA-polymerase	Gibco BRL, Karlsruhe
Temed	Roth, Karlsruhe
TGFß1	R&D, Minneapolis, USA
Tris	Roth, Karlsruhe
Trypan blue	Biochrom AG, Berlin
Trypsin-EDTA	Gibco BRL, Karlsruhe
XhoI	NEB, Frankfurt a. M.

4.1.1 Kits

Apoptag® Peroxidase	Millipore, Schwalbach
In Situ Apoptosis Detection Kit	
CD326+ (EpCAM) Isolation Kit	Miltenyi Biotec, Bergisch Gladbach
CD56+ T Cell Isolation Kit	Miltenyi Biotec, Bergisch Gladbach
CD8+ T Cell Isolation Kit	Miltenyi Biotec, Bergisch Gladbach
Cell proliferation ELISA, BrdU	Roche, Mannheim
CytoTox 96 Non-Radioactive	Promega, Mannheim
Cytotoxicity Assay	
Dual-Luciferase Reporter Assay System	Promega, Mannheim
M30-Apoptosense® ELISA	Peviva, Bromma, Sweden
Naïve CD4+ T Cell Isolation Kit	Miltenyi Biotec, Bergisch Gladbach
Phototope® HRP Western Blot Detection Kit	Cell Signaling, NEB, Frankfurt a. M.
QIAquick Gel Extraction Kit	Qiagen, Hilden
RNeasy Mini-Kit	Qiagen, Hilden
SuperScript First-Strand Synthesis	Gibco BRL, Karlsruhe
System for RT-PCR	

4.2 Media, buffers and solutions

4.2.1 Media

DMEM 10% FCS	DMEM	
	FCS	10%
	pyruvate	1 mM
	gentamycin	50 µg/ml
DMEM 5% CCS	DMEM	
	CCS	5%
	pyruvate	1 mM
	gentamycin	50 µg/ml

CCS: Charcoal and sulfatase treated FCS for

	cell culture experiments:	
	500 ml FCS is incubated with 2 U/ml sulfatase at 37°C and heatinactivated two times for 30 min at 56°C	
DMEM 10% human AB serum	DMEM	
	human AB serum	10%
	pyruvate	1 mM
	gentamycin	50 µg/ml
LB medium	bacto trypton	1% w/v
	yeast extract	0.1% w/v
	NaCl	0.2 mM
	ampicillin	50 µg/ml
	adjust to pH 7.0	
organ transport medium	Liforlab®	
	colistin	100 µg/ml
Freezing medium	DMEM	
	FCS	20%
	DMSO	10%
SOC	trypton	2%
	yeast extract	0.5%
	NaCl	10 mM
	KCl	2,5 mM
	MgCl2	10 mM
	MgSO4	10 mM
	glucose	20 mM

4.2.2 Buffer

10x PCR buffer	Tris-HCl, pH 8.8	100 mM
	KCl	500 mM
	$MgCl_2$	15 mM
	gelatine	0.01% (w/v)
10x cell lysis buffer	Tris-HCl pH 7.6	200 mM
	NaCl	1.5 mM
	EDTA	10 mM
	EGTA	10 mM
	Triton X-100	10%
	sodium phosphate	25 mM
	Na_3VO_4	10 mM
	Leupeptin	10 µg/ml
Cell Rinse buffer	NaCl	120 mM
	Glucose	15.6 mM
	$MgCl_2$ x $6H2O$	2.5 mM
	KCl	5.4 mM
	NaH_2PO_4	1 mM
	HEPES	20 mM
	adjust to pH 7.2	
MACS buffer	PBS	
	EDTA	2 mM
	BSA	0.5%
Transfer buffer	Tris	48 mM
	glycin	39 mM
	SDS	0.037%
	methanol	20%
	adjust to pH 9.1	

TBS 10 x	NaCl	1.45 M
	KCl	25 mM
	Tris	250 mM
	adjust to pH 7.4 with HCl	

TBST 1 x	1:10 dilution of 10 x TBS-concentrate	
	+ Tween 20	0.2%

Running buffer 10x	Tris	250 mM
	glycin	2 M
	SDS	10%

Stripping solution	SDS	0.2%
	ß-mercaptoethanol	400 μl
	1 x TBS	ad 50 ml

Laemmli buffer 5x	Tris-HCl	312.5 mM
	glycerol	25%
	SDS	10%
	bromophenol blue	0.05%
	ß-mercaptoethanol	25%
	adjust to pH 6.8	

4.2.3 Solutions

4-hydroxytamoxifen	10^{-4} M in 96% ethanol
APS 10%	1 g ammonium peroxide disulfate
	ad. 100 ml aq. dest.
ICI 182.780	10^{-6} M in 96% ethanol
Interleukin-2	100 μg/ml in 20 mM acetic acid
Propidium iodide	50 μL PI, 10 μl RNase A (=1 mg) in 950 μl
	PBS 1% glucose
SDS 10%	10 g sodium dodecyl sulfate
	ad 100 ml aq. dest.

TGFß1	10 ng/µl in 4 mM HCl, 0.1% BSA
Tris-HCl 0.5 M	30 g Tris-(hydroxymethyl)-aminomethan,
	adjust to pH 6.8 with conc. HCl
	aq. dest ad 500 ml
Tris-HCl 1.5 M	90.75 g Tris-(hydroxymethyl)-aminomethan,
	adjust to pH 8.8 with conc. HCl
	aq. dest ad 500 ml

4.2.4 Cell lines

MCF-7 cells were received from the national cancer institute (NCI, Bethesda, Maryland, USA) and served as a model for human estrogen receptor positive (ER+) mammary carcinoma. The mink lung cell line CCL64 was kindly provided by Prof. Dr. L. Graeve (University of Hohenheim) and was used to establish a reporter gene based TGFß bioassay.

E. coli INVα´ bacteria (Invitrogen, Germany) were employed for plasmid amplification.

4.3 Primer, plasmids and antibodies

4.3.1 Primer for quantitative LightCycler RT-PCR

name	sequence 5' ⇨3'
FasL as	TGC CAG CTC CTT CTG TAG GT
FasL se	GGC CTG TGT CTC CTT GTG AT
Foxp3 as	TGG GAA TGT GCT GTT TCC AT
Foxp3 se	TGA CCA AGG CTT CAT CTG TG
GATA-3se	AAG GCT GTC TGC AGC CAG GA
GATA-3 as	AGG GGT CTG TTA ATA TTG TGA AGC TTG T
GzmA as	AGC AGG GTC TCC GCA TTT AT
GzmA se	CCT CCG AGG TGG AAG AGA CT
GzmB as	GCC ATT GTT TCG TCC ATA GC
GzmB se	GGA AGA TCG AAA GTG CGA AT
GUS as	ATG CCC TTT TTA TTC CCC AGC
GUS se	GCT CAT TTG GAA TTT TGC CG
PRF1 as	AGT GTG TAC CAC ATG GAA ACT GTA G

PRF1 se	GCA ATG TGC ATG TGT CTG TGG CC
RORγt se	ACA GAG ATA GAG CAC CTG GT GCA G
RORγt as	ACA TCT CCC ACA TGG ACT TCC TCT
Tbet se	ATG CCA GGA AAC CGC CTG TA
Tbet as	GGA GCA CAA TCA TCT GGG TCA CAT T

4.3.2 Sequencing primer

name	sequence 5' ⇨3'
pCB7-1 as	TTA TAC AGG GCG TAC ACT TTC
pCB7-1 se	TGG TTG GAA AAT GGA GAA GA
pCB7-2 as	TTA AAA ACA TGT ATC ACT TTT
pCB7-2 se	TAT GAC CAT CTT CTG TAT TC

4.3.3 Plasmids

p3TP-lux	TGFß responsive reporter plasmid based on pGl3-Basic (Wrana *et al.*, 1992)
p6SBE	TGFß reporter plasmid with 6 copies of the Smad binding element (5'-GTCTAGAC-3') based on the pGl3-Promoter vector (Le Dai *et al.*, 1998)
pCB7-1IrNeo	a pCMViresNeo derived expression vector containing a neomycin resistance gene and the human B7-1 (CD80) gene under control of the *cytomegalovirus* (CMV) promoter (University of Halle)
pCB7-2IrNeo	a pCMViresNeo derived expression vector containing a neomycin resistance gene and the human B7-2 (CD86) gene under control of the *cytomegalovirus* (CMV) promoter (University of Halle)
pGL3-Promoter	reporter plasmid containing the *firefly luciferase* gene without promoter (Promega, Mannheim)
pGl3-Basic	reporter plasmid containing the *firefly luciferase* gene under control of a SV40 promoter (Promega, Mannheim)
pHRL-TK	control plasmid to determine transfection efficacy, contains the *renilla luciferase* gene under control of the *Herpes simplex* thymidine kinase promoter (Promega, Mannheim)

4.3.4 Primary antibodies

anti ß-actin	mouse IgG1, monoclonal, Sigma, Taufkirchen
anti B7-1	mouse IgG1, monoclonal, Santa Cruz biotechnology, Heidelberg
anti B7-2	mouse IgG1, monoclonal, Santa Cruz biotechnology, Heidelberg
anti CD28	mouse IgG1, monoclonal, BD Pharmingen, Heidelberg
anti CD3	mouse IgG1, monoclonal, BD Pharmingen, Heidelberg
anti FasL	rabbit, polyclonal, New England BioLabs® GmbH, Frankfurt
anti GAPDH	BIODESIGN international® and OEM Concepts Brands, Saco, ME USA
anti GzmB	mouse IgG1, monoclonal, Santa Cruz biotechnology, Heidelberg
anti PRF1	rabbit IgG, polyclonal, Santa Cruz biotechnology, Heidelberg

4.3.5 Secondary antibodies

anti mouse	goat IgG-HRP, monoclonal, Santa Cruz biotechnology, Heidelberg
anti rabbit	goat IgG-HRP, monoclonal, Santa Cruz biotechnology, Heidelberg

4.3.6 Neutralizing antibodies

anti TGFß1	mouse IgG1, monoclonal, R&D systems, Wiesbaden
anti TGFß2	goat IgG, polyclonal, R&D systems, Wiesbaden
anti TGFß1, 2, 3	mouse IgG1, monoclonal, R&D systems, Wiesbaden

4.3.7 Equipment

Agarose gel chamber	B1A	PeqLab, Erlangen
Bacteria shaker	HAT	Infors, Bottmingen
Blotting chamber	Fast-Blot B33	Biometra, Göttingen
Brightfield microscope	ID03	Zeiss, Jena
Centrifuges	Biofuge fresco	Heraeus, Fellbach
	Universal 320 R	Hettich, Tuttlingen
CO_2 incubator	Hera cell 150	Heraeus, Hanau
Confocal laser scanning microscope	Leica DM IRBE	Leica Lasertechnik, Wetzlar

Counting chamber	Neubauer improved	Roth, Karlsruhe
Electroporator	Easyject plus	Peqlab, Erlangen
ELISA reader	Wallac Victor 1420	Wallac, Perkin Elmer, USA
Flow cytometer	FACScan	Becton Dickinson, USA
Luminometer	Autolumat plus	Berthold, Bad Wildbach
Spectrophotometer	Nanodrop ND-1000	Peqlab, Erlangen
Pipettes	0.1-2.5µl, 0.5-10µl, 10-100 µl, 200-1000 µl	Eppendorf, Hamburg
Power supplies	Power Pac P25 (Fast-Blot)	Biometra, Göttingen
	Power Pac 3000 (PAGE)	BioRad, München
	E143 (agarose gels)	
Software	GraphPad Prism	GraphPad Software Inc., San Diego, USA
Sterile bench	BSB 4A	Gelaire, Sydney, Australia
Thermo-cycler	LightCycler	Roche, Mannheim
	Mastercycler Gradient	Eppendorf, Hamburg
Tissue slicer	Krumdieck Tissue Slicer	Krumdieck, Alabama Research and Development Corp., Munford, USA

5 METHODS

5.1 Cell culture (cell lines)

5.1.1 Cultivation of cell lines

MCF-7 cells as well as the mink lung line CCL64 were grown at 37°C in 5% CO_2 atmosphere in DMEM containing 4.5 g glucose/liter supplemented with 50 µg/ml gentamicin, 1 mM sodium pyruvate and 10% fetal calf serum (FCS). Both adherent cell lines were passaged twice a week by removal of the supernatants, a washing step with PBS and subsequent application of trypsin-EDTA. After detachment of cells, fresh medium was added and the cell suspensions were distributed to new flasks. Prior to experiments including AE treatment or cocultivation with AE treated cells, cell culture medium was changed to DMEM (supplemented as above) with 5% charcoal stripped serum (CCS) instead of FCS until the next passage.

5.1.1.1 Cryopreservation

For cryopreservation confluent cells were washed in PBS, trypsinized, counted and adjusted to a concentration of 10^6/ml in freezing medium consisting of DMEM with 10% DMSO and 20% FCS. Cryotubes were filled each with 1 ml of the cell suspension and stored at -20°C for 24 h. Afterwards they were transferred to -80°C for at least 24 h and finally stored in a nitrogen tank. As needed, cells were thawed in a 37°C waterbath and quickly washed in fresh medium prior to cultivation.

5.1.2 Stable transfection of MCF-7 cells

The effectene tranfection kit from Quiagen was used for stable transfections. In a first step, a buffer and the so called enhancer solution lead to the condensation of the utilized plasmid DNA. The addition of effectene causes spontaneous formation of micelles which can cross cell membranes due to their lipophilic properties.

MCF-7 cells were grown in DMEM 5% CCS for one passage. The nearly confluent cells were trypsinized, seeded in 6 well plates in a concentration of $5x10^4$ cells per well and incubated over night. The next day the transfection mix containing 400 ng of plasmid DNA was prepared following the manufacturer´s instructions. Application on the adhered MCF-7 cells followed. After two days of incubation, 400 µl of trypsin-EDTA was added on the cells of each well subsequently to removal of the supernatant and a washing step with PBS. After losing adherence, the cells from each well were distributed on 2 100 mm Ø petri dishes containing 10 ml DMEM

10% FCS and 800 µg/ml G418 for selection of successfully transfected cells. The concentration of G418 was adjusted to an amount, which only allowed growth of cells with stably integrated expression plasmids. G418 supplemented medium was changed every 3 days. After a week, macroscopically visible colonies occurred and their location was additionally labeled at the bottom of the dish. Supernatants were discharged, cells were washed in PBS and small plastic cylinders with silicone grease on the lower brim were fixed above the colonies. The plastic cylinders were filled with 100 µl of trypsin-EDTA to detach the cells of the chosen colony. After carefully repeated pipetting, the cells were transferred into a cavity of a 24-well plate containg 1 ml of fresh DMEM 10% FCS supplemented with 800 µg G418. Cultivation in T 25 cell culture flask followed.

5.1.2.1 FACS analysis of transfected cellsurface molecules

To confirm a successful transfection and the resulting expression of cellsurface molecules, a FACS analysis was performed. 10^6 cells from each clone were blocked in 100 µl PBS 1% BSA for 10 min followed by the application of 1 µg of the specific antibody or 1 µg of isotype control antibodies, respectively. After 30 min of incubation at 4°C, cells were washed in 1 ml PBS 1% BSA and resolved in 100 µl PBS 1% BSA. Then 0.5 µg of a FITC conjugated secondary antibody was added for another incubation of 30 min at 4°C. Finally, cells were washed, resuspended in 1 ml PBS 1% BSA and assessed in a flow cytometer.

5.1.2.2 Detection of transfected surface molecules by fluorescence microscopy

Stably transfected MCF-7 cells were cultivated on 8 compartment chamber slides. In each chamber 4×10^4 cells were seeded in a volume of 300 µl DMEM 10% FCS with 800 µg/ml G418 and incubated at 37°C until 50% of confluency was reached. The supernatant was removed and the cells were fixed on the slide during 5 min of incubation in icecold 100% ethanol at -20°C. To wash the cells PBS was added 2 times for 5 min. Then a blocking step followed by adding PBS 1% BSA for 45 min at room temperature. Afterwards, the primary antibody was applied in a 1:100 dilution for 1 h. Subsequently, the cells were washed 2 times in PBS 1% BSA followed by incubation with the FITC-labeled secondary antibody for 1 h at room temperature. Finally, the cells were washed 3 times for 5 min and cover slides were fixed with a mounting solution for fluorescence microscopy.

5.1.3 Transient transfection of CCL64 cells

To establish a TGFß sensitive bioassay, the mink lung cell line CCL64 was transfected with p3TP-lux, a TGFß responsive reporter plasmid containing the firefly luciferase gene. Electroporation was used for transfection.

To this, $4x10^6$ cells were resuspended in 400 µl DMEM 5% CCS and transferred to a 4 mm electroporation cuvette. 15 µg/ml of p3TP-lux was added to the cell suspension. The same concentration of promotorless vector pGL3-Basic was used as control. For normalization to transfection efficiency both plasmids were cotransfected with 4 µg/ml of the renilla luciferase gene containing pHRLTK vector. After a minute of incubation with the plasmid DNA, the cuvettes were fixed in the electroporator and a single pulse program (250 V, 1800 µF) was conducted for transfection. Afterwards, the 400 µl cell suspension from each cuvette were quickly diluted in 20 ml DMEM 5% CCS.

5.1.3.1 Quantitative TGFß bioassay

To quantify the amount of secreted bioactive TGFß in cell supernatants p3TP-lux/pHRLTK or pGL3-Basic/pHRLTK transfected CCL64 ($7x10^4$/well) were cocultivated with MCF-7 cells or primary tumor cells in a final volume of 1 ml medium per cavity on 24-well plates for 24 hours. Subsequently, the supernatants were taken off and the adhered cells were washed with 1 ml PBS per well. 100 µl *passive lysis buffer* was added and the cell culture plates were placed on a shaker for 15 min at room temperature. Cell lysates were mixed by pipetting and 40 µl were transferred into luminometer tubes. Afterwards, the measurement was performed on a luminometer (*Autolumat Plus*, Berthold Technologies, Bad Wildbad, Germany) using the *dual luciferase® reporter assay system* (Promega). Automatic application of 50 µl *luciferase assay reagent II* (*LAR II*) was used for determination of firefly luciferase. In a second step 50 µl 1x stop and glow reagent was automatically added. Thereby, firefly luciferase activity was stopped and renilla luciferase enzymatic activity was detected instead of.

A standard curve was created by treating transfected CCL64 cells with increasing amounts (5 pM to 100 pM) of human isolated TGFß1 and TGFß2 (R&D), respectively. Concentrations of secreted bioactive TGFß in cocultures were determined by extrapolation.

5.2 Cell culture (primary cells)

5.2.1 Primary blood cells

Blood was obtained from healthy female donors. Peripheral blood mononuclear cells (PBMC) were harvested by means of *Ficoll* (Biochrom AG, Berlin, Germany) based density gradient centrifugation at 1400 rpm for 25 min. Buffy coats were taken off and washed 2 times in PBS 2 mM EDTA. In case of a leukopheresis surplus PBMCs were deep frozen in DMEM containing 10% DMSO and 20% FCS. Thawed PBMC were maintained in DMEM containing 4.5 g glucose/liter supplemented with 50 µg/ml gentamicin, 1 mM sodium pyruvate and 5% CCS for one day prior to usage in experiments.

5.2.2 Isolation of T cell subsets

For the isolation or depletion of lymphocyte subpopulations, magnetic cell separation technology MACS (Miltenyi Biotec, Bergisch Gladbach, Germany) was employed according to the manufacturer´s instructions. Cytotoxic T lymphocytes were selected using CD8 antibody coated magnetic beads. Naïve CD4+ T helper cells were negatively selected. Anti CD56 beads were used for the isolation or depletion of NK cells. For direct treatment with antiestrogens, lymphocytes were cultivated in DMEM 5% CCS.

5.2.3 Cultivation of primary mammary carcinoma tissue slices

Only samples from patients who agreed to a consent form were included in this study. Tissue from large (> 3 cm) and untreated mammary carcinoma was directly received after surgery, trimmed in the pathology lab of the Robert-Bosch-Hospital and kept on ice in *Liforlab*® culture medium with 100 µg/ml colistin. Afterwards, cylindrical pieces with a radius of 5 mm were punched out under sterile conditions. A precision cutting tissue slicer (Krumdieck, Alabama Research and Development Corp., Munsford, USA) was used to cut 0.2 mm thick slices, which were collected in sterile PBS with 50 µg/ml gentamycin. Tissue slices were then cultivated in 96- or 24-well plates in DMEM containing 4.5 g glucose/liter and supplemented with 10% human AB serum (Invitrogen), 50 µg/ml gentamicin and 1 mM sodium pyruvate. After 24 h treatment with either 1 µl/ml 100% ethanol, 10^{-9}M ICI 182.780 or 10^{-7}M 4-hydroxytamoxifen started for 5 days.

5.2.4   Isolation of EpCAM + primary tumor cells

A scalpel was used to cut the part of the tumor tissue, which remained after the punshing procedure, into small pieces. These pieces were dissociated during 1.5 hours of incubation in an enzyme-cocktail consisting of a protease (0.25 mg/ml), a DNase (250 U/ml) and a collagenase (167 U/ml) (Sigma, Taufkirchen, Germany) at 37°C. Subsequently, the suspensions were applied on a nylon filter with a pore width of 30 µm to obtain single cells. Epithelial tumor cells were isolated using the *EpCAM+ cell isolation kit* (Miltenyi) following the instructions of the manufacturer. For cultivation of tumor cells 96- or 24-well plates (Nunc) were coated with 2% collagen IV in sterile PBS for at least 30 min at room temperature. Cells were kept in 100 µl DMEM 10% human AB serum in case of 96-well cell culture plates and in 1 ml per well on 24-well plates. After 24 h treatment with 1 µl 100% ethanol, 10^{-7} M 4-hydroxytamoxifen or 10^{-9} M fulvestrant followed for 5 days.

5.2.4.1   TUNEL staining of EpCAM+ tumor cells

After the autologous MLTR, tissue slices from the same treatment were pooled and EpCAM+ cells were isolated as described above. Also EpCAM+ cells, which were isolated from the start and cultivated in 96-well cell culture plates, were trypsinized and collected after the removal of effector cells from MLTR. The detection of apoptosis followed. To this, isolated tumor cells from each treatment were resuspended in 100 µl PBS for subsequent cytospins. Cell death measurement was detected in a TUNEL assay according to the instructions of the producer (Millipore). Briefly, double strand breaks, which indicate late apoptotic events, were elongated with digoxigenin labeled nucleotides by means of a terminal deoxynucleotidyl transferase. Enzyme coupled digoxigenin antibodies were incubated on the cytospins and addition of DAB substrate led to a colorimetric reaction. Lightmicroscopical photos were made for documentation and counting, which was performed by two independent investigators.

5.2.5   Isolation and cultivation of tumor infiltrating lymphocytes

On the day of arrival, tumor infiltrating lymphocytes (TIL) were also isolated from single cell suspensions of dissociated tumor tissues. For this purpose, the *CD3+ T cell isolation kit* (Miltenyi) was employed. Isolated TIL were cultivated in T25 cell culture flasks using 10 ml DMEM 10% human AB serum as medium. For reactivation of TIL 0.1 µg/ml interleukin-2 (Immunotools, Friesoythe, Germany) was added each 24 h for 4 days. One day prior to the MLTR, they were additionally activated with 1 µg/ml plate bound CD3 antibody and 1 µg/µl soluble CD28 antibody. To gain sufficient numbers of cells for the following MLTR, TILs were pooled with activated autologous PBMC.

5.3 Cocultures, MLC and MLTR

5.3.1 Insert based cocultures

MCF-7 cells were seeded in 24-well plates with each well containing $2x10^4$ cells in 1ml DMEM 5% CCS. After 24 h, medium was renewed and antiestrogens were added in the concentrations of 10^{-9}M ICI 182.780 and 10^{-7}M OHT, respectively. These growth inhibitory but sublethal concentrations were detemined by dose response curves (data not shown). On day 3 of antiestrogen treatment, lymphocyte subpopulations were isolated as described above. For activation of lymphocytes cell culture inserts (0.8 µm pore, Nunc, Langenselbold, Germany) were coated with PBS containing 0.5 µg/ml CD3 antibody (R&D, Wiesbaden, Germany) at 37°C for 1 h. Subsequently, the inserts were placed upon the treated MCF-7 cells and $8x10^5$ lymphocytes in 100 µl DMEM 5% CCS containing 10 µg/ml soluble CD28 antibody (R&D) were added. 3 µg/ml of a panspecific TGFß antibody was used for neutralization of antiestrogen induced TGFß (R&D). CD8+ and CD4+ T cells were harvested for RNA and/or protein isolation after 48 and 72 h, respectively.

5.3.1.1 Suppressor assay and BrdU ELISA

CD4+ T cells from MCF-7 cell cocultures were pooled with autologous naïve CD4 T cells in a 1:1 ratio ($5x10^4$ each) and seeded in 96-well plates, which were coated with PBS containing 0.5 µg/ml CD3 antibody (R&D). The final volume was 100 µl DMEM 5% CCS containing 10 µg/ml soluble CD28 antibody (R&D). After 4 days, BrdU was added for 24 h and a BrdU ELISA (Roche, Mannheim, Germany) was performed as described by the producer. Briefly, cells were fixed and DNA was denatured for better accessibility of incorporated BrdU. After incubation with an enzyme coupled BrdU antibody, TMB substrate is added for colorimetric detection in an ELISA reader.

5.3.2 Mixed lymphocyte culture

PBMC from 2 different healthy female donors were isolated by means of *Ficoll* gradient centrifugation as described above. $2x10^6$ PBMC from both individuals were pooled in 24-well cell culture plates in a final volume of 1 ml DMEM 10% human AB serum per well for 4 days. 10 µM BrdU was added 16 h prior to the end of the reaction. 10 pM of human TGFß1 was used.

5.3.2.1 FACS analysis for detection of BrdU incorporation

After 4 days of cocultivation including 16 h of BrdU incubation, the cells were washed in 1 ml PBS 1% BSA and centrifuged. The pellet was carefully resuspended in icecold 70% ethanol by cautious vortexing and the suspensions were stored at -20°C over night for fixation of cells. Afterwards, the cells were slowly resuspended in 1 ml 2N HCl 5% Triton X-100 for 30 min of DNA denaturation. Borax was used to neutralize the acid and cells were washed and suspended in 100 µl PBS 1% BSA, 0.5% TWEEN. Incubation with 1 µg BrdU antibody for 30 min at 4°C followed. After a washing step, the cells were again resuspended in 100 µl PBS 1% BSA, 0.5% TWEEN and 0.5 µg of a FITC-labeled secondary (goat-anti-mouse) antibody was applied for 30 min at 4°C. Cells were stained in 1 ml propidium iodide solution with RNase A and assessed in FACS analysis.

5.3.3 Heterologous mixed lymphocyte tumor reactions

MCF-7 cells were seeded in 96-well plates applying 10^4 cells per well in 100 µl DMEM 5% CCS. The next day, antiestrogen treatment followed for 4 days (concentrations as indicated for the coculture assay). On day 4, non activated PBMC from healthy female donors were freshly isolated and added in a 10:1 effector to target cell ratio. For this purpose, a triplet of wells with MCF-7 cells from each treatment was trypsinized and cell numbers were determined in a counting chamber. Alternatively, natural killer (NK) cells were depleted from PBMC using the *CD56+ cells isolation kit* (Miltenyi). PBMC without NK cells were also applied in a 10:1 ratio as opposed to NK cells alone. As their actual percentage in the PBMC population is about 10% a 1:1 effector to target cell ratio was chosen for MLTR with NK cells. The final reaction volume was 110 µl DMEM 5% CCS in each well. After 24 hours of coincubation, LDH release in the supernatants was measured as an indicator of cell death.

In a modification of this approach, a preincubation step was added. MCF-7 cells were seeded in 6-well plates applying $5x10^5$ cells per well in 2 ml DMEM 5% CCS. AE were added after 24 hours. On day 2 of treatment $5x10^6$ PBMC were added for 4 days and taken off subsequently to be applied on freshly seeded MCF-7 cells in 96-well plates. Effector to target cell ratios and cell death measurement were retained. A panspecific TGFß neutralizing antibody (R&D) was used during both MLTR in a concentration of 10µg/ml.

5.3.3.1 LDH release measurements

After 24 hours of coincubation, plates were centrifuged and supernatants were collected. To determine resulting cell death of MCF-7 cells, LDH release was measured using the *CytoTox 96 Non-Radioactive Cytotoxicity Assay* (Promega, Mannheim, Germany) following the manufacturer´s instructions.

5.3.3.2 Cytokine arrays

MCF-7 cells were seeded in 6-well plates with a concentration of 5×10^5 cells in 2 ml DMEM 5% CCS per well. After 24 h, treatment with either ethanol, fulvestrant or 4-hydroxytamoxifen followed for 2 days. PBMC were applied in a 10:1 ratio for another 4 days. Alternatively, MCF-7 cells were cultivated for 6 days as described but without application of PBMC. Subsequently, supernatants were collected and cytokine array analyses (Biocat, Heidelberg, Germany) were performed according to the manufacturer´s instructions. The protein array (RayBio® *Human Cytokine Antibody Array 3*) comprised 40 common cytokines.

5.3.4 Autologous MLTR

Slices and tumor cells were cultivated on collagen IV-coated 96-well plates in 200 µl DMEM 10% human AB serum per well for 6 days in total. Treatment with 1 µl/ml ethanol, 10^{-7} M 4-hydroxytamoxifen or 10^{-9} M fulvestrant started 24 h after cultivation start for 5 days. Isolated TIL were reactivated with interleukin-2 from the first day. On day 4, blood was obtained from the same patient and PBMC were isolated as described above. Both IL-2 stimulated TIL and autologous PBMC were pooled to reach sufficient cell numbers in the MLTR. Aditionally, they were activated on 24-well cell culture plates with 1 µg/ml plate bound CD3 antibody and 1 µg/µl soluble CD28 antibody 24 h prior to the MLTR on day 5 to day 6. After activation, 10 µl medium including 10^6 TIL/PBMC were added on each tumor slice resulting in a final volume of 210 µl. Numbers of adherent EpCAM+ tumor cells per well were determined and activated TIL/PBMC were applied in 10:1 ratio. After 24 hours of MLTR, immune cells in the supernatant were collected. Slices from each treatment were pooled and dissociated as described above. CD3+ TILs and EpCAM+ tumor cells were isolated using the MACS system. mRNA levels in lymphocytes were assessed with real time PCR and tumor cells were fixed on cover slides using a cytospin centrifuge. Apoptosis was measured afterwards with the TUNEL assay as described above.

5.4 Nucleic acid analysis and preparation

5.4.1 RNA isolation

RNA isolation was performed using the *RNeasy Mini Kit* (QIAGEN, Hilden, Germany). Lysates from $8x10^5$ to 10^6 lymphocytes were mixed with equal volumes of 70% ethanol and applied onto columns. Washing steps and an incubation with a DNase followed according to manufacturer´s instructions. Afterwards, 30 μl of nuclease free water were used for eluation of retained RNA. Concentration was determined using a *nanodrop* spectrophotometer (PeqLab).

5.4.2 cDNA synthesis

RNA was reversely transcribed into cDNA by means of the *SuperScript First-strand-synthesis system* for RT-PCR (Invitrogen). 100 to 250 ng/μl of total RNA were used for the reaction. Partially, RNA solutions had to be concentrated in a speed vac centrifuge.

5.4.3 Quantitative real time PCR (*light cycler*)

Quantitative real time PCR is based on the same principles as the common PCR. Moreover, fluorescent dyes like *SybrGreen*, which intercalate with double-stranded DNA, can be added. The interaction with double-stranded DNA leads to an increase of emitted fluorescence from the dye and can therefor be used for quantification of newly synthesized amplicon DNA after each cycle of the PCR. Standard DNA samples of the appropriate target gene were used in each run for absolute quantification by generating a calibration line for subsequent extrapolation. Standard DNA was produced in a PCR with the same primers and conditions as in the actual qRT-PCR. The product was applied on a 1% agarose gel for confirmation of expected size and the PCR *purification kit* (Qiagen) was used for isolation of DNA. Subsequently, the concentration was detemined on a nanodrop spectrophotometer and the solution was aliquoted. 1:10 dilutions from 100 fg to 10 ag were freshly prepared for each qRT-PCR run to enable extrapolation of absolute values from a calibration line.

Each qRT-PCR program started with a denaturation step at 95°C for 2 seconds followed by 40 amplification cycles (temperature transition rate of 20°C/second). Annealing was performed at 60°C (FasL, T-bet, GATA-3, RORγt), 63°C (GUS), 66°C (GzmB, Foxp3) and 69°C (PRF1) for 8 sec, each followed by an elongation phase for 10 sec at 72°C. cDNA was applied either undiluted (FasL, Foxp3, GUS PRF1) or in a 1:10 dilution (GzmA, GzmB).

	final concentration	volume [µl]
H_2O		2.34
5x PCR buffer	1x	2
dNTP (2.5 mM)	250 µM	1
se primer (10 µM)	0.2 µM	0.2
as primer (10 µM)	0.2 µM	0.2
$MgCl_2$ (50 mM)	3 mM	0.6
BSA 0.1%	0.01%	1
SybrGreen 1:1000 (Roche)		0.5
Taq pol 5U/µl (Invitrogen)	0.8 U	0.16
cDNA	2.0 µl	

5.4.4 Transformation of competent E.coli

E.coli were used for the *in vivo* amplification of plasmid DNA. To this, 50 µl of competent INVαF′ cells were thawed on ice and 10-100 ng DNA were added. After 30 min of incubation on ice, a heat shock followed for 40 sec at 42°C to enable the uptake of plasmid DNA into bacteria cells. Afterwards, cells were quickly cooled on ice for 2 min and 250 µl of SOC medium was added for 1 h of incubation in a 37°C shaker. Subsequently, suspensions were distributed on ampicillin containing (0.1 mg/ml) LB agar plates and incubated over night at 37°C.

5.4.5 Preparation of plasmid DNA from bacteria

Colonies were picked and incubated in LB medium (50 µg/ml ampicillin) in a 37°C shaker over night. The *maxi-plasmid purification kit* from Qiagen was employed for isolation of plasmid DNA according to the instructions of the producer. Briefly, bacteria were lysed and DNA was denatured in an alkaline buffer. Neutraliziation of the lysate results in the exclusive solution of DNA in the liquid phase, which can be separated by centrifugation. Afterwards, columns are used for purification and retained plasmid DNA was eluted in H_2O. The DNA concentrations were determined by means of a *nanodrop* spectrophotometer from PeqLab.

5.4.6 Restriction enzyme digestion

Restriction enzymes were used to characterize expression vectors. The inserted DNA sequence was cut out at specific regocnition sites. Different units of restriction enzymes data (mostly 5 units per µg DNA) and adequate buffers were used according to the manufaturer′s instructions.

The reaction volume was adjusted to 20 µl with H$_2$O followed by incubation for 1 h at 37°C. Afterwards, the product was applied on a 1% agarose gel for detection of resulting fragment sizes.

5.5 Protein preparation and analysis

5.5.1 Protein isolation and quantification

Lymphocytes (8×10^5-10^6) from cocultivation with AE treated MCF-7 cells (see above) were lysed in 50 µl 1x cell lysis buffer supplemented with 1 mM PMSF and 1% protease inhibitor cocktailset (Calbiochem, Darmstadt, Germany) for 30 min on ice. Afterwards, lysates were centrifuged at 13,000 rpm for another 30 min at 4°C. Supernatants were collected and Bradford staining was performed for quantification. To this, a calibration line was generated by solving different amounts of BSA in a range of 1-16 µg/ml in 20% *Bradford* reagent. The actual specimens were dissolved in an equal volume of *Bradford* reagent. After 5 min of incubation, absorbance was measured in a spectrophotometer (Hewlett-Packard, Waldbronn) at a wave length of 595 nm.

5.5.2 Electrophoretic separation on SDS-PAGE

Samples were denatured at 95°C for 5 minutes after addition of *Laemmli* buffer containing SDS, which renders all proteins negatively charged for better separation in subsequent electrophoresis. Furthermore, the destruction of three dimensional structures of the proteins is enhanced by ß-mercaptoethanol, which breaks disulphide bonds. Afterwards, the denatured protein samples were applied on SDS-PAGE with either 8% of acrylamide for big proteins (50-200 kDa) or 12% for small proteins (10-60 kDa). Gels for SDS-PAGE consisted of stacking and separating gels.

	stacking gel (4%)	separating gel (8%)	separating gel (12%)
30% acrylamide/BIS	2.0 ml	8.0 ml	12.0 ml
0.5 M Tris pH 6.8	3.8 ml	-	-
1.5 M Tris pH 8,8	-	7.5 ml	7.5 ml
10% SDS	150 µl	300 µl	300 µl
H$_2$O	9.2 ml	13.9 ml	9.9 ml
TEMED	15 µl	18 µl	12 µl
10% APS	150 µl	300 µl	300 µl

Electrophoresis was conducted for 3.5 h at 170 V in 1x electrophoresis buffer.

5.5.3 Western blot

Semidry electrophoretic transfer of separated proteins from acrylamide gels to a protein binding nitrocellulose membrane was achieved by voltage application using a *fast blot* transfer chamber (Whatman). Between the plate electrodes, a sandwich consisting of 2 blotting papers, the protein gel, a nitrocellulose membrane and another 2 blotting papers was applied and soaked with transfer buffer. Blotting followed for 15 min at 400 mA.

5.5.4 Western blot analysis

To avoid unspecific binding of primary antibodies, western blot membranes were incubated in TBST 5% skim milk powder for 1 h at room temperature. After 3 times of washing in TBST for 5 min, primary antibodies were incubated over night at 4°C except the ß-actin antibody (1 h at room temperature) in the following dilutions: GzmB 1:500, PRF1 1:200, FasL 1:500 and ß-actin 1:5000. Again, the blots were washed 3 times and secondary peroxidase conjugated antibodies were added for 1 h at 4°C. Final washing (3 times for 5 min in TBST) was accomplished to get rid of unbound secondary antibody solution. Subsequently, the *Pierce*® *ECL Western Blotting Substrate* (Thermo scientific) was used for detection in a Fuji *Image Reader LAS-1000*. Analysis was performed with the *Aida* software (version 3.21; Raytest, Straubenhardt). For detection of proteins with similar molecular weights, the western blot membranes were stripped in stripping solution for 30 min at 56°C and anewly incubated with primary and secondary antibodies as described above.

5.6 Statistics

At least 3 independent experiments were used to calculate mean values ± standard errors of the mean. Standard deviations smaller than 0.5% are not shown. Statistical analysis like unpaired t tests was performed with the *GraphPad Prism* software. P values < 0.05 were considered as significant (* < 0.05; ** < 0.01; *** < 0.001).

6 RESULTS

6.1 Antiestrogen induced TGFß – preliminaries for the coculture system

It has been shown in our group that antiestrogen treatment leads to the activation of the TGFß system in the breast cancer cell line MCF-7 (Knabbe, 1987). The mRNA levels of the ligand TGFß2 as well as the TGFß receptor type II were elevated by the application of ICI 182.780 and 4-hydroxytamoxifen. Besides, enhanced secretion and activation of TGFß1 was observed. To test whether the increase of bioactive TGFß in the extracellular space suffices to inhibit effector T cells and to induce the conversion of naïve CD4 T cells into regulatory T cells, cocultures with antiestrogen treated MCF-7 cells were established.

6.1.1 Dose depedent downregulation of CD8 T cell effector molecules by TGFß1

First of all, the impact of isolated human TGFß1 (R&D) on the transcriptional regulation of crucial effector molecules in CD8+ T cells was determined in dose dependency experiments followed by qRT-PCR. This approach was chosen to elucidate the amounts of TGFß1, which could possibly lead to inhibition of effector functions, as seen by downregulation of GzmA, GzmB, FasL and PRF1. To this, PBMC from healthy donors were used for the isolation of CD8+ cytotoxic T cells by means of the MACS technology. CD8+ T cells were then suspended in DMEM 5% CCS and seeded on 24-well plates in the concentration of $8x10^5$ to 10^6 cells in 1 ml per well. Simultaneous to activation with CD3 and CD28 antibodies, different concentrations of human TGFß1 in a range from 1 pM to 300 pM were applied in dublicates. To maintain isolated TGFß1 in its bioactive form and preventing it from binding to the latency associated protein, 4 mM HCl 0.1% BSA served as vehicle and was also used as control treatment of each experiment. Figure [1A] shows the intense TGFß1 responsiveness of GzmB mRNA regulation. Only 1 pM TGFß1 suffices to reduce the GzmB mRNA expression level to 75%. The following concentrations ranging from 3 to 1000 pM result in a constant expression level at about 50% of control without further downregulation. GzmA mRNA expression tends to a more linear downregulation pattern due to increasing amounts of TGFß1. 10 pM TGFß1 are necessary to reach 75% of control and 50% reduction of GzmA mRNA expression levels is not achieved until a concentration of 1000 pM TGFß1 is applied

[Fig 1B]. The dose dependent effects of TGFß1 on FasL mRNA results in a transcriptional regulation pattern resembling the one seen for GzmB. As little as 1 pM TGFß1 suffices to reduce the FasL mRNA level to three-fourth of controls. Higher concentrations from 3 to 1000 pM caused the FasL mRNA expression to settle down at about 50% of control with a slight increase at 1000 pM [Fig.1C]. 1 pM of TGFß sufficed to decrease PRF1 mRNA levels to 50% of control. The TGFß concentrations, which followed, resulted in a strong inhibition, keeping the expression at about 30% of the untreated control [Fig. 1D].

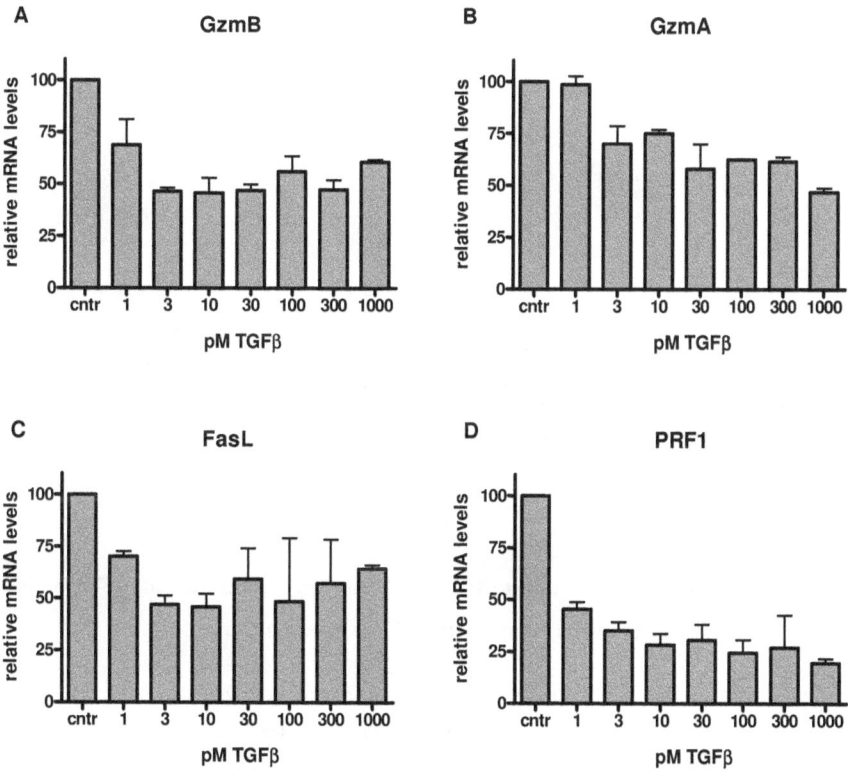

Figure 1. Downregulation of effector molecules in CD8+ T cells after TGFß treatment

A)-D) show effector molecule mRNA expression in CD3/CD28 antibody activated CD8+ T cells after treatment with increasing concentrations of TGFß. PBMC were obtained from healthy female donors and CD8+ T cells were isolated using the MACS system. After 48 h of TGFß treatment, RNA was isolated, transcribed into cDNA and effector molecule mRNA expression levels were measured in qRT-PCR.

6.1.2 Dose depedent induction of Foxp3 in naïve CD4+ T cells by TGFß1

A similar approach as for cytotoxic effector molecules in CD8+ T cells was used for determination of dose dependent effects of TGFß1 on mRNA expression of the transcription factor Foxp3 in naïve CD4+ T cells. After isolation naïve CD4+ T cells were seeded on 24-well plates ($4x10^5$ to 10^6 per well) in DMEM 5% CCS and activated via CD3/CD28 antibodies. TGFß1 in different concentrations was added simultaneously to activation. Interestingly, the increasing amounts of TGFß1 used in this assay (3-300 pM) did not lead to a plateau in Foxp3 mRNA levels. The expression did not level off at a certain percentage as seen for GzmB or PRF1 but continuously mounted from a 1.2-fold increase in case of 5 pM TGFß1 to a 27-fold induction when a concentration of 400 pM TGFß1 was applied [Fig.2].

FoxP3

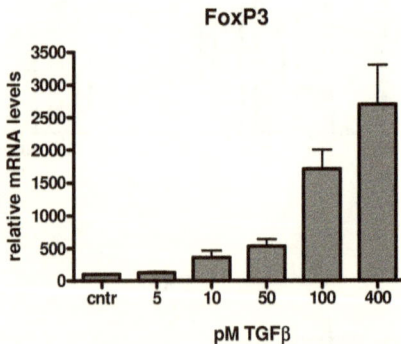

Figure 2. Induction of Foxp3 in naïve CD4+ T cells

Naïve CD4+ T cells were isolated from blood of female donors and activated via CD3/CD28 antibodies. Simultaneously, TGFß was applied in different amounts. After 48 h Foxp3 mRNA levels were assessed in qRT-PCR.

6.1.3 Establishment of a quantitative TGFß bioassay/ Quantification of bioactive TGFß in antiestrogen treated MCF-7 cell supernatants

After elucidating the TGFß sensitivity of cytotoxic effector molecule and Foxp3 mRNA, regulation in activated CD8+ and CD4+ T cells, respectively, the amounts of bioactive TGFß in supernatants of antiestrogen treated MCF-7 cells had to be determined. For this purpose, the mink lung cell line CCL64, which is known to be highly sensitive to TGFß was used for transfection of the TGFß responsive reporter gene plasmid p3TP-lux. Activation of TGFß signaling leads to expression of the firefly luciferase gene, which can be quantified by application of the adequate substrate and luminometric measurement in a subsequent luciferase assay. A second vector containing a renilla luciferase gene under a constitutively active promoter was cotransfected for normalization to transfection efficiency.

MCF-7 cells were seeded in 24-well plates and treated with ethanol, 10^{-9} M ICI 182.780, or 10^{-7} M 4-hydroxytamoxifen for 4 days. At that time, CCL64 were transfected with the reporter plasmids and promotorless control vectors via electroporation. Afterwards, they were directly seeded on top of the treated MCF-7 cells. This coculture was harvested after 24 h of incubation by lysis of the adhered cells and luciferase measurement was performed. In parallel, transfected CCL64 cells were treated with different amounts of TGFß1 in a range of 1 to 100 pM. This approach was processed equally to the MCF-7 cell cocultures for generation of a calibration line from which the amounts of TGFß in the supernatants of MCF-7 cells were extrapolated. Luciferase activity in the directly treated, non-cocultivated CCL64 showed a steady rise in the range from 3 to 10 pM TGFß1 allowing for linear extrapolation [Fig.3A]. Cocultivations revealed a basal secretion/presence of about 4 pM/ml bioactive TGFß in the supernatants of ethanol treated MCF-7 cells. Furthermore, cocultures with ICI 182.780 treated MCF-7 cells resulted in a 3-fold increase of luciferase activity compared to control indicating an augmentation from 4 to approximately 10 pM/ml TGFß. A 2-fold increase to about 8 pM of bioactive TGFß was reported for 4-hydroxytamoxifen treated MCF-7 cells [Fig.3B]. The application of conditioned medium from antiestrogen treated MCF-7 cells on transfected CCL64 resulted in very weak luciferase signals. Moreover, there was no increase in comparison to the ethanol treated control (data not shown). This phenomenon, which seemed to happen during centrifugation is probably due to the rapid binding of active TGFß to the latency associated protein (> 2 min) in the supernatants without constant reactivation by MCF-7 cells. As a consequence, only inactive/latent TGFß is assessed in the assay.

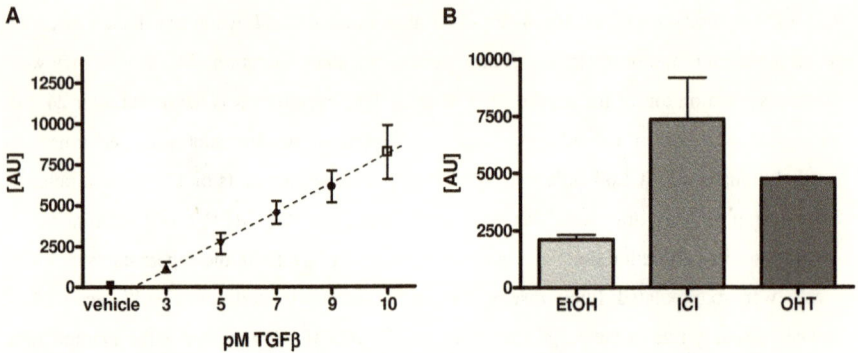

Figure 3. Quantification of TGFß in MCF-7 cell supernatants after antiestrogen treatment

The mink lung cell line CCL64 was transiently transfected with the luciferase gene containing TGFß reporter plasmid p3TP-lux and control vectors. Electroporation was used. A) Transfected cells were seeded in 24-well plates and treated with different amounts of human TGFß1 for 24 h to generate a calibration line. Luciferase activity was assessed in a luminometer. B) MCF-7 cells were cultivated on 24-well plates and antiestrogens were applied for 4 days. CCL64 cells were electroporated with the reporter vector and directly seeded on the treated MCF-7 cells. After 24 h of coculture, luciferase activity was measured and TGFß1 amounts were extrapolated from the calibration line.

6.2 Cocultures

6.2.1 Antiestrogen treated MCF-7 cells downregulate cytotoxic effector molecule mRNA expression in activated CD8+ T cells

After clarifying the amounts of bioactive TGFß in antiestrogen treated MCF-7 cell supernatants and the effects of different TGFß concentrations on the transcriptional regulation of effector molecules in CD8+ T cells, cocultures of both cell types were carried out. To this, MCF-7 cells were cultivated in 24-well plates and ethanol, ICI 182.780 or 4-hydroxytamoxifen was applied for 3 to 4 days. Cytotoxic CD8+ T cells were isolated from different healthy female blood donors using the MACS system (Miltenyi). Activation via CD3/CD28 antibodies followed in cell culture inserts, which were employed for MCF-7 cell cocultivation to create a double chamber system where cells are separated by a membrane allowing exchange of soluble mediators. By using this approach, activation of T cells coincided with the start of the coculture. After 48 h of coincubation, cytotoxic T cells were harvested, RNA was isolated and transcribed into cDNA, which was assessed in qRT-PCR. MCF-7 cell treatment with both ICI 182.780 and 4-hydroxytamoxifen led to a significant decrease of mRNA expression for GzmB, PRF1 and FasL in CD8 T cells to 50% of ethanol treated control [Fig. 4]. To affirm the crucial role of antiestrogen induced TGFß in these cases, a panspecific TGFß neutralizing antibody was applied. Its ability to reverse the effector molecule downregulation was shown [Fig.4A, C, E]. The regulation of GzmA in CD8+ T cells from MCF-7 cell cocultures showed a high variability between different blood donors. In this case no significant downregulation was observed (data not shown).

To rule out direct effects of antiestrogens on the transcriptional regulation of effector molecules, activated CD8+ T cells were separately treated with ICI 182.780, 4-hydroxytamoxifen or TGFß1 as a positive control. In this case no MCF-7 cells were present. Subsequent qRT-PCR showed no alteration of mRNA levels of GzmB, FasL and PRF1 when antiestrogens were applied. In contrast, TGFß1 strongly reduced the expression of these molecules to about 30% of control [Fig.4B, D, F]. GUS mRNA levels were used for normalization in all qRT-PCRs.

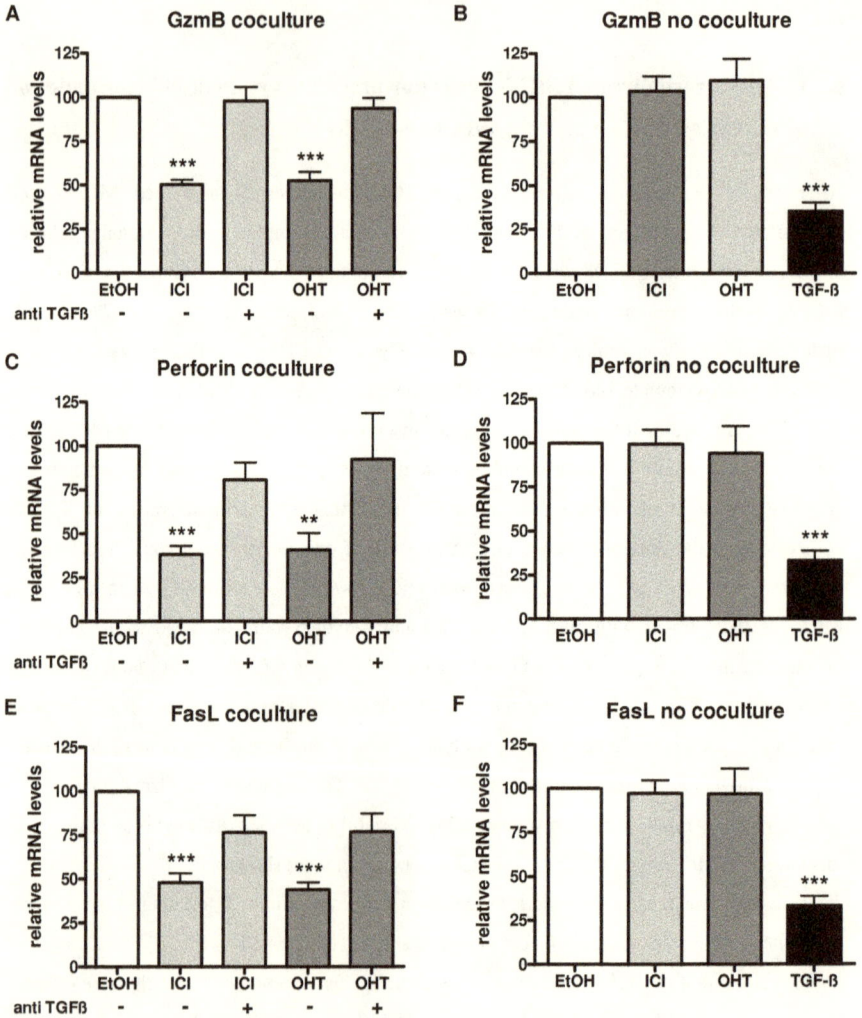

Figure 4. Downregulation of effector molecules in CD8+ T cells in coculture with AE treated MCF-7 cells

A), C) and E) show effector molecule mRNA expression in CD3/CD28 antibody activated CD8+ T cells after an insert based cocultivation with ethanol versus 10^{-7} M 4-hydroxytamoxifen or 10^{-9} M ICI 182.780 treated MCF-7 cells. The downregulation in the presence of AE was reversed by addition of a panspecific TGFß neutralizing antibody. The data represent mean ± SD from 5 experiments, each with duplicates. In B), D) and F) isolated and activated human CD8+ T cells were treated with either ethanol, AE or 10^{-11} M human TGFß1 for 2 days.

6.2.2 Western blot analysis of CD8+ T cells effector molecules after cocultivation with antiestrogen treated MCF-7 cells

CD8+ T cell/MCF-7 cell cocultures as described above were also used to monitor changes in cytotoxic protein levels due to application of antiestrogens. CD8+ T lymphocytes were lysed after 48 h of coincubation with antiestrogen treated MCF-7 cells and western blot analysis for GzmB and PRF1 was performed. ß-actin was used for normalization [Fig.5A, B]. The decrease in protein signals caused by antiestrogen treatment of MCF-7 cells was reversible with a TGFß neutralizing antibody. Despite testing of several antibodies from different sources, none was found to be suitable for the detection of FasL.

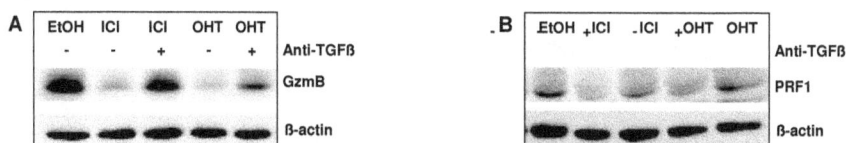

Figure 5. Downregulation of effector molecules in CD8+ T cells in coculture with AE treated MCF-7 cells

A and B show representative western blot analysis of effector molecule protein expression in CD3/CD28 antibody activated CD8+ T cells after an insert based cocultivation with ethanol versus 10^{-7} M 4-hydroxytamoxifen or 10^{-9} M ICI 182.780 treated MCF-7 cells. The downregulation in the presence of AE was reversed by addition of a panspecific TGFß neutralizing antibody. ß-actin was used as a control in the western blots.

6.2.3 Antiestrogen treated MCF-7 cells induce Foxp3 mRNA expression in activated naïve CD4+ T cells

Another lymphocyte population of interest is the CD4+ T cell subset. CD4+ T cells can be converted into immunosuppressive regulatory T cells in the presence of TGFß. A hallmark for this differentiation is the induction of the transcription factor Foxp3. The established cocultivation system was employed to scrutinize the ability of antiestrogen treated MCF-7 cells to cause upregulation of Foxp3 mRNA. MCF-7 cells were cultivated and treated in 24-well plates and naïve CD4+ T cells were isolated on day 3. Activation via CD3/CD28 antibodies followed in cell culture inserts together with the start of the coculture. After 3 days lymphocytes were lysed and RNA levels were assessed in qRT-PCR. Application of ICI 182.780 on MCF-7 cells prior to the cocultivation led to a 2.5-fold increase in Foxp3 mRNA expression. A 3-fold induction was seen for 4-hydroxytamoxifen treatment. Again, the TGFß specificity of these effects were proven by addition of a panspecific TGFß neutralizing antibody, which inhibited Foxp3 mRNA level elevation during antiestrogen treated cocultures [Fig.6A].

A direct participation of antiestrogens on the transcriptional regulation of this transcription factor had to be excluded. For this purpose, naïve CD4+ T cells were activated and separately treated with ICI 182.780 or 4-hydroxytamoxifen without the presence of MCF-7 cells. Again, TGFß application was used as a positive control and resulted in 2.5-fold increase in Foxp3 mRNA expression. Similar TGFß concentrations as determined in antiestrogen treated MCF-7 cell supernatants were used [Fig.6B].

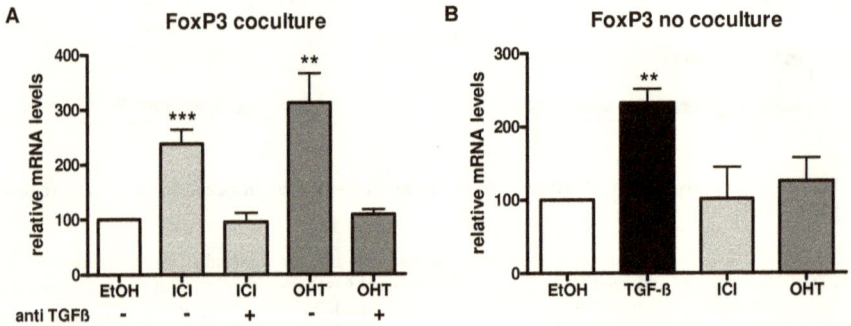

Figure 6. Induction of Foxp3 in naïve CD4+ T cells

A) RT-PCR measurement of Foxp3 mRNA expression in CD3/CD28 antibody CD4+ T cells after an insert based cocultivation with ethanol versus AE (concentration see Fig.3) treated MCF-7 cells. The induction in the presence of AE was reversed by addition of a panspecific TGFß neutralizing antibody. The data represent mean ± SD from 5 experiments, each with duplicates. B) Isolated and activated human CD4+ T cells were treated with either ethanol, AE or 10^{-11} M human TGFß1 for 3 days.

6.2.4 CD4+ T cells from antiestrogen treated cocultures exhibit suppressive potential

It has been reported that Foxp3 can be transiently upregulated in activated CD4+ lymphocytes without leading to differentiation into regulatory T cells (). We therefore assessed the functional activity of Foxp3+ CD4+ T cells induced in antiestrogen stimulated MCF-7 cocultures in a suppressor assay. To this, the induced Tregs were transferred in a 1:1 ratio to cultures of freshly isolated CD4+ lymphocytes from the same donor and the coculture was treated with CD3 and CD28 specific antibodies for T cell activation to occur. Cell proliferation was measured at day 5 by BrdU incorporation. In the Foxp3+ coculture, proliferation was found to be reduced to 50% (4-hydroxytamoxifen) or 75% (ICI 182.780) of controls, indicating that cocultivation of naïve CD4+ cells with antiestrogen treated MCF-7 cells had generated functional Foxp3+ Treg cells [Fig. 7].

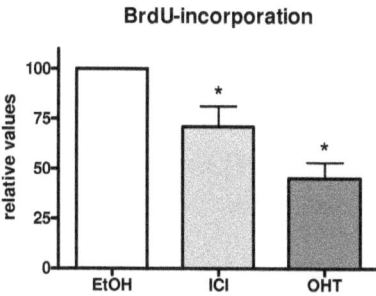

BrdU-incorporation

Figure 7. CD4+ T cells from MCF-7 cocultures and their suppressive potential

CD4+ T cells from cocultures with antiestrogen treated MCF-7 cells were applied in a suppressor assay with freshly isolated autologous CD4+ T cells for 5 days. Subsequently, a BrdU ELISA was performed.

6.3 TGFß completely inhibited proliferation in mixed lymphocyte cultures

As so far only artificially activated and isolated T cell subsets were employed in the experimental setting of this work, an approach, which allows for predication of TGFß effects on the entire immune cell network was chosen. Mixed lymphocyte cultures permit the usage of complete PBMC populations and constitute a model system of T cell activation without dependency on stimulating antibodies or mitogens. PBMC of 2 different donors were pooled and BrdU was added on day 4 for 24 h. Due to differences in the MHC of both individuals a mutual rejection occurred. The intensity of the emerging immune response is indicated by the incorporation of BrdU into freshly synthesized DNA during proliferation of participating lymphocytes. FACS analysis was used to detect BrdU uptake into the cells genomes. In Fig.8 BrdU incorporation in PBMC after a mixed lymphocyte culture is shown. Separated cells from both donors were used as control. In comparison to separated immune cells from donor A or B, there is a 3-fold enhancement of proliferation when PBMC from both donors were pooled. The concomitant application of TGFß completely inhibited this increase. The amount of applied TGFß was similar to that determined in antiestrogen treated MCF-7 cell supernatants by the CCL64 cell bioassay.

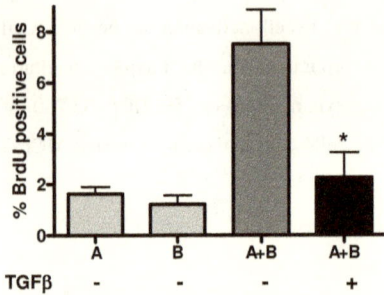

Figure 8. Effect of TGFß on PBMC proliferation in a mixed lymphocyte culture

PBMC from 2 different donors were isolated. On either separated or pooled PBMC (+/-TGFß) BrdU was applied after 5 days for 24 h. FACS analysis was performed to measure BrdU incorporation as an indicator for proliferation.

6.4 Heterologous mixed lymphocyte tumor reactions

So far, the role of antiestrogen induced TGFß from MCF-7 cells on cytotoxic lymphocyte effector molecule transcription and CD4+ T cell differentiation was shown in a two chamber cocultivation system. Besides, exogenously added TGFß in mixed lymphocyte cultures strongly inhibited the onset of an immune response, normally emerging from the encounter of 2 different PBCM populations. To gain insights in the effects of antiestrogen induced TGFß from MCF-7 cells on the function of immune cells, a mixed lymphocyte tumor reaction was established. Like the mixed lymphocyte culture this approach allows for the utilization of the entire PBMC population and the abandonment of artificial activation.

6.4.1 Preliminary experiments with activated cytotoxic CD8+ T cells

To optimize the mixed lymphocyte tumor reaction and the subsequent read out, an approach, which guarantees a robust response was chosen. The usage of activated CD8+ lymphocytes should circumvent the interindividual variety in cytotoxic potential. At the same time, the employed effector cells should be susceptible enough to monitor effects of antiestrogen induced TGFß in MCF-7 cells. In a first step, different ratios of effector to target cells were tested to determine a proportion resulting in stable cytotoxicity without using excessive numbers of lymphocytes. Besides, the percentage of resultant cell death should allow for modulation by TGFß into both directions without reaching the limit of detection.

MCF-7 cells were cultivated in 96-well plates for 1 day, CD8 T cells were isolated and activated over night. On the next day, different ratios of effector to target cells were prepared. After 24 h supernatants were collected and an LDH assay was carried out. Fig.9A shows the augmentation of the percentage of dying cells when increasing numbers of activated cytotoxic T cells were used. The exogenous addition of TGFß during CD3/CD28 activation strongly decreased the killing potential of CD8+ T cells in the subsequent mixed lymphocyte tumor reaction [Fig.9B].

To see wether antiestrogen induced TGFß suffices to impair cytotoxicity of CD8+ T cells, MCF-7 cells were seeded in 24-well plates. After 24 h of incubation, treatment with ethanol or ICI 182.780 was conducted for 4 days. In parallel, cytotoxic lymphocytes were isolated, activated over night and applied onto treated MCF-7 cells on day 4. After 24 h, cell death was assessed in a LDH assay, which showed a reduction of cytotoxicity to a fourth of control [Fig.9C].

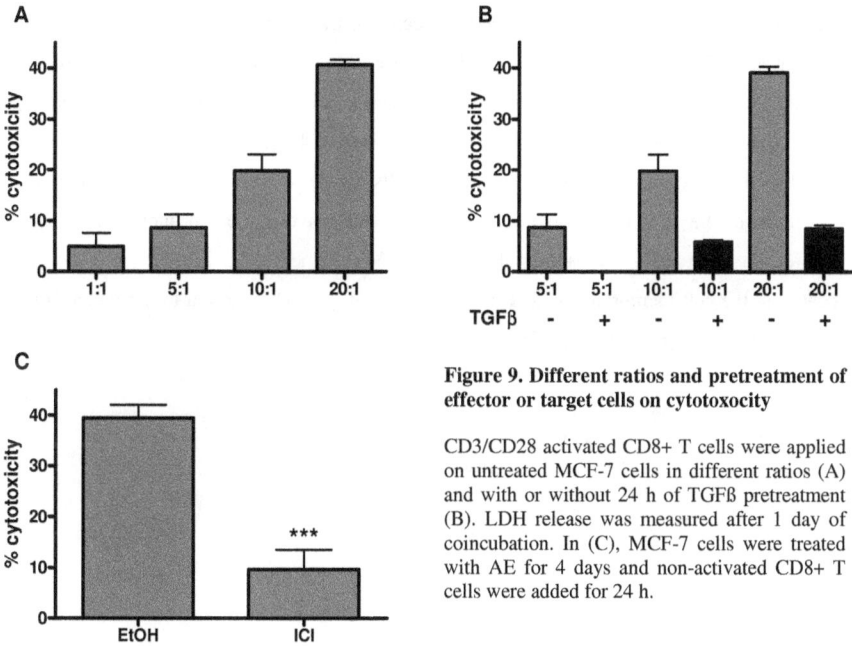

Figure 9. Different ratios and pretreatment of effector or target cells on cytotoxocity

CD3/CD28 activated CD8+ T cells were applied on untreated MCF-7 cells in different ratios (A) and with or without 24 h of TGFß pretreatment (B). LDH release was measured after 1 day of coincubation. In (C), MCF-7 cells were treated with AE for 4 days and non-activated CD8+ T cells were added for 24 h.

6.4.2 Stable B7-1 and B7-2 transfection of MCF-7 cells – a tool for effector cell stimulation

As absolute values of mRNA expression levels in lymphocytes from insert based cocultures greatly differed between blood donors, a high variability of cytotoxic potential in the MLTR was also expected. To countervail this putative problem, MCF-7 cells were stably transfected with the T cell costimulatory molecules B7-1 and B7-2. These proteins are normally expressed on antigen presenting cells like dendritic cells and serve as ligands for the CD28 receptor on T cells, which provides auxiliary activation stimuli in addition to T cell receptor signaling.

B7-1 and B7-2 expression vectors containing a G418 selection marker were amplified in bacteria and transfected into MCF-7 cells. Successful transfection was shown via antibody staining in FACS analysis. Additionally, the proper location of the membrane proteins B7-1 and B7-2 was determined by means of fluorescence microscopy after antibody staining. Fig.10A shows analysis of one representative clone out of 4, respectively. It became evident that the atopic expression of B7-2 in MCF-7 cells seems to work better then in the B7-1 transfection. The shift of positive cells in FACS analysis was more pronounced for B7-2 transfectants. Besides, microscopy showed antibody stained B7-2 proteins to be clearly located in the cell membranes with a more distinct signal in comparison to the rather grainy pictures of B7-1 expression [Fig.10B].

A   **B**

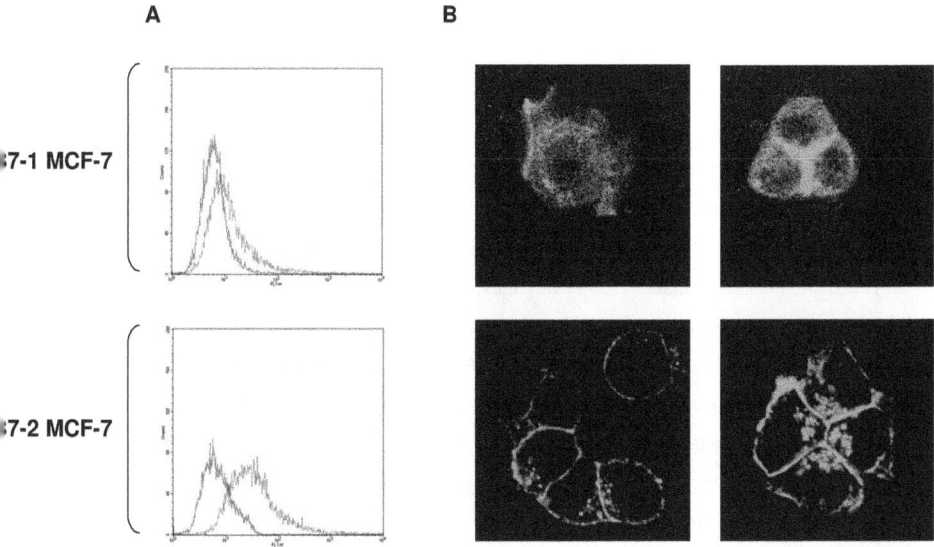

Figure 10. Stable transfection of MCF-7 cells with B7-1 and B7-2 expression vectors

MCF-7 cells were stably transfected with either B7-1 or B7-2 expression plasmids containing a G418 resistance gene. After cultivation in selection medium, clones were picked and analyzed for proper expression. A) Specific antibodies (left curves) were used for subsequent FACS analysis including an IgG control (right curves). B) After incubation with specific primary and FITC labeled secondary antibodies fluorescence microscopy was used to assess localization of B7-1 or B7-2 protein on transfected MCF-7 cells.

6.4.3 Mixed lymphocyte tumor reactions with B7-1 and B7-2 transfected MCF-7 cells

To test whether the B7-1 and B7-2 expressing MCF-7 cells own the potential to enhance cytotoxicity and even stimulate non-activated lymphocytes during a mixed lymphocyte tumor reaction, the transfectants were cultivated on 96-well plates for 24 h. In parallel, CD8+ T cells from healthy female donors were isolated. For the following mixed lymphocyte tumor reaction, T cells were either activated or cultivated in DMEM 5% CCS over night. The next day, activated or unstimulated CD8+ lymphocytes were added on the adherent target cells in a 10:1 ratio. After 24 h, LDH measurement was performed.

In accordance with the differences in B7-1 and B7-2 protein expression and location in MCF-7 cells, a different stimulation of cytotoxicity was observed. Unlike B7-1 transfectants, B7-2 expressing MCF-7 cells succeeded in boosting the killing activity of unstimualted CD8+ T cells to a level, which is comparable to that seen in controls with activated lymphocytes [Fig.11A]. Next, MCF-7 wildtype cells and those transfected with T cell costimulatory molecules were compared. This time, only B7-2 transfectants were used due to their more adequate characteristics. Besides, MCF-7 target cells were treated with ethanol or ICI 182.780 for 4 days. Non-activated CD8+ T cells were applied in a ratio of 10:1 and cytotoxicity was measured 24 h later in a LDH assay. In Fig.11B, the interindividual variability of cytotoxic responses is exemplarily demonstrated based on the results from 2 different donors. Lymphocytes from donor A exhibited a strong response at about 40% of cytotoxicity independent of B7-2 expression. Antiestrogen treatment of target cells led to an intense diminution of killing. In comparison, CD8+ T cells from donor B showed a lower cytotoxicity against both B7-2 transfected and wildtype MCF-7 cells. However, the B7-2 transfectant caused a 2-fold increase in killing. Antiestrogen treatment of both target cell lines led to a similar decrease of cytotoxicity.

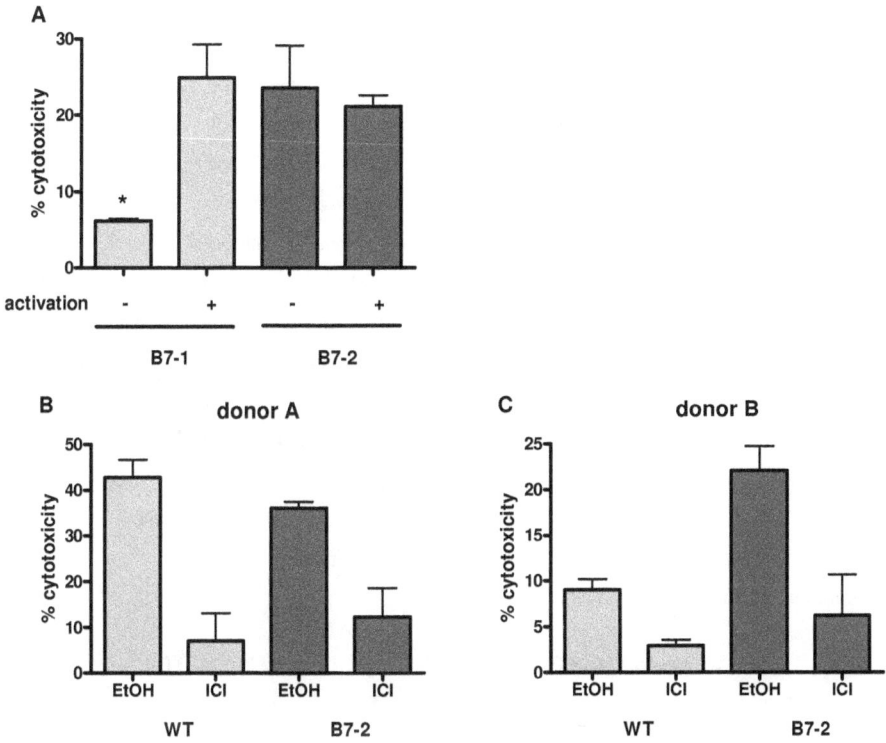

Figure 11. Mixed lymphocyte tumor reactions with B7-1 and B7-2 transfectants

Stably transfected MCF-7 cells were used as target cells in a heterologous mixed lymphocyte tumor reaction with unstimulated or CD3/CD28 antibody activated CD8+ T cells in a 10:1 ratio. After 24 h, supernatants were collected for LDH measurement. In A), the potential of transfectants to enhance cytotoxicity of unstimulated CD8+ T cells was compared. Activated lymphocytes served as positive control. B) and C) show the interindividual differences in mixed lymphocyte tumor reactions with wildtype and B7-2 transfected MCF-7 cells. Target cells were cultivated and ICI 182.780 was applied for 4 days. Unstimulated CD8 T cells were added in a 10:1 ratio and LDH release was measured after 24 h.

6.4.4 Mixed lymphocyte tumor reactions with wildtype MCF-7 cells

As tranfection with costimulatory molecules failed to even out varying response intensities of lymphocytes from different donors, wildtype MCF-7 cells were used for the following experiments. To calculate significances, only relative values from single experiments were used for statistics. In order to account for the complexity of the anti-tumor immune response the entire PBMC population was employed. Furthermore, artificial activation was avoided.

MCF-7 cells were treated with antiestrogens for 4 days. PBMC from healthy female donors were directly added to the MCF-7 monolayer and LDH release from tumor cells was measured 24 hours later as a benchmark for cytotoxic effector cell activity. To preclude any direct impacts of antiestrogens on the functionality of immune cells, PBMC were pretreated for 24 hours with antiestrogens and added to untreated MCF-7 target cells [Fig. 12A]. In this case, no reduction of cytotoxic activity was detected. However, on antiestrogen treated MCF-7 cells, cytotoxic activity of effector cells was strongly reduced (25% and 40% of control for ICI and OHT, respectively) [Fig. 12B]. This inhibition was reversed when a TGFß neutralizing antibody was present during the MLTR, proofing that TGFß mediates the inhibition of cytotoxic effector cell generation.

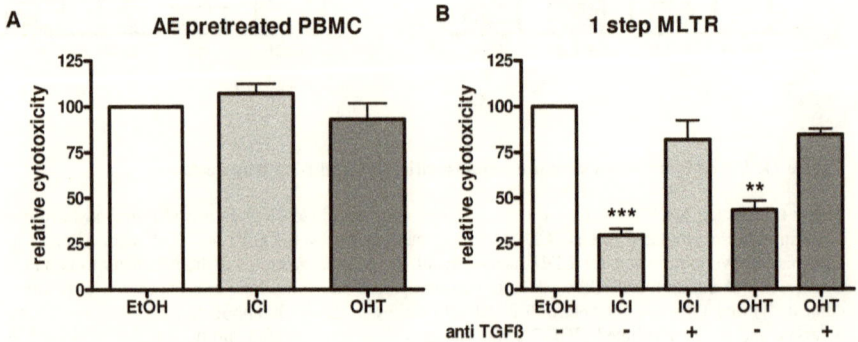

Figure 12. Antiestrogen treatment of effector or target cells in heterologous mixed lymphocyte tumor reactions

A) To test whether antiestrogens have a direct impact on the cytotoxicity of immune cells, PBMC were isolated and pretreated with ethanol, ICI 182.780 or 4-hydroxytamoxifen for 24 h. In parallel, wildtype MCF-7 cells were cultivated on 96-well plates over night without any treatment. Lymphocytes were applied in the ratio of 10:1 and LDH release was measured after 24 h. In B), MCF-7 cells were treated with ethanol or antiestrogens for 4 days. PBMC were isolated and directly added without pretreatment and LDH release was measured 24 h later. The decrease of cytotoxicity seen in antiestrogen treatment could be reversed by addition of a panspecific TGFß neutralizing antibody.

6.4.4.1 Innate immunity – the role of NK cells during the heterologous mixed lymphocyte tumor reaction

To elucidate the participation of NK cells within the population of cytotoxic effector cells in freshly isolated PBMC, NK cells were depleted by CD56 beads. Their absence in PBMC caused a 50% decrease of cytotoxicity [Fig. 13A]. The activity of purified NK cell was found to be equally sensitive to inhibition by the antiestrogen induced TGFß in the mixed lymphocyte tumor reaction, as shown by reversibility with the neutralizing antibody [Fig. 13B]. Fulvestrant (ICI) reduced the cytotoxixcity of NK cells to 30% and 4-hydroxytamoxifen (OHT) led to a decrease to about 40% of control.

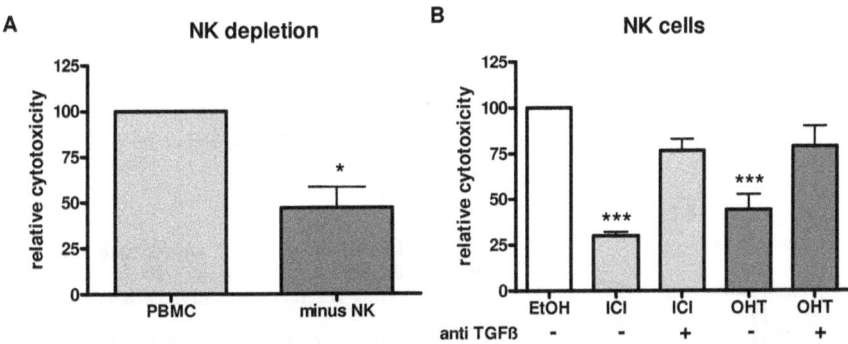

Figure 13. Participation of NK cells in heterologous mixed lymphocyte tumor reaction and NK cells sensitivity to TGFß

A) To test the participation of NK cells on cytotoxicity seen in the mixed lymphocyte tumor reaction, they were depleted from PBMC using anti-CD56 MACS beads prior to application on untreated MCF-7 cells. After 24 h, LDH release was measured. B) Target MCF-7 cells were treated with antiestrogens for 4 days to test the sensitivity of NK cells to induced TGFß. NK cells were isolated and applied in a 1:1 ratio for 24 h. A neutralizing antibody was used for confirmation of TGFß specific effects.

6.4.4.2 Adaptive immunity – clonal expansion of specific lymphocytes on antiestrogen treated MCF-7 cells impaired effector cell functions

Furthermore, the inhibitory action of antiestrogen induced TGFß from MCF-7 cells on the induction of antigen specific cytotoxic effector cells was determined. To this, a preincubation step was inserted in the course of the MLTR model described above. PBMC were isolated and coincubated with antiestrogen treated MCF-7 cells on 6-well plates for 5 days in a 10:1 ratio. This approach allows for priming and expansion of MCF-7 specific cytotoxic T cells. Afterwards, supernatants containing immune cells were collected, whereas MCF-7 cells remained adhered to the surface of the cell culture plates. Effector cells were washed, counted and their activity was determined in a subsequent cytotoxicity assay on untreated MCF-7 cells.

The generation of cytotoxic T lymphocytes (CTL) was greatly diminished when antiestrogens were present during the activation phase [Fig. 14]. CTL generation was nearly completely restored when the neutralizing TGFß antibody was present during the activation period.

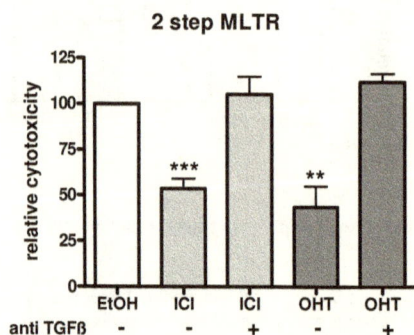

Figure 14. Effect of antiestrogen treatment during a heterologous mixed lymphocyte tumor reaction with a preincubation step

Ethanol or AE treated MCF-7 cells and PBMC were co-incubated for 4 days. Subsequently, suspension cells were collected, lymphocytes were counted and applied in an MLTR with non treated MCF-7 cells (10:1). The TGFß neutralizing antibody was added during the preincubation step.

6.4.5 T helper cell differentiation during a heterologous mixed lymphocyte tumor reaction

The varying differentiation of T helper cells can skew an immune response against pathogens or malignant cells into several directions, including cell directed Th1 responses, humoral Th2 responses and Th17 lymphocyte based reactions in inflammation. As these processes largely depend on the present cytokine composition, protein arrays comprising 40 common cytokines and subsequent real time PCR, assessing Th cell subset specific transcription factors were accomplished.

6.4.5.1 Protein arrays of secreted cytokines did not show alterations after antiestrogen treatment

To rule out the influence of antiestrogen regulated cytokines on immune cells during the heterologous mixed lymphocyte tumor reaction, protein array analyses were performed. Cytokine secretion from MCF-7 cells alone and from ethanol or antiestrogen treated mixed lymphocyte tumor reactions was determined and compared. The mixed cultures of PBMC plus MCF-7 cells [Fig. 15A1-A3] led to increased signals (compared to MCF-7 cells alone, Fig. 15 B2) for IL-6, IL-10 and IL-13, typical Th2 response and suppressive cytokines, which are thought to promote tumorigenesis. Furthermore, monocyte chemotactic protein-2 and -3 (MCP-2/-3), epithelial neutrophil activating peptide-78 (ENA-78) and growth regulated oncogene-α (GRO-α) were also detectable when MCF-7 cells and PBMC were pooled. However, compared to ethanol treatment [Fig. 15A1] addition of fulvestrant [Fig. 15A2] or 4-hydroxytamoxifen [Fig. 15A3] did not lead to significant alterations of the mentioned cytokines. To determine background signals, which derive from the used cell culture medium, DMEM 5% CCS was also assessed in the cytokine array analysis. Very low levels of IL-10 and the chemotactic protein RANTES (regulated upon activation, normal T-cell expressed and secreted) were deteceted [Fig. 15B1]. The array only detects active TGFß. Due to TGFßs rapid reversion into its latent form during processing of supernatants, no signal could be measured. Acid activation of TGFß was not suitable with regard to detection of other cytokines, which do not require activation and may be structurally altered by such a procedure.

	a	b	c	d	e	f	g	h	i	j	k	l
1	Pos	Pos	Neg	Neg	ENA-78	GCSF	GM-CSF	GRO	GRO-α	I-309	IL-1α	IL-1ß
2	Pos	Pos	Neg	Neg	ENA-78	GCSF	GM-CSF	GRO	GRO-α	I-309	IL-1α	IL-1ß
3	IL-2	IL-3	IL-4	IL-5	IL-6	IL-7	IL-8	IL-10	IL-12p40p70	IL-13	IL-15	IFNγ
4	IL-2	IL-3	IL-4	IL-5	IL-6	IL-7	IL-8	IL-10	IL-12p40p70	IL-13	IL-15	IFNγ
5	MCP-1	MCP-2	MCP-3	MCSF	MDC	MIG	MIP-1δ	RANTES	SCF	SDF-1	TARC	TGF-ß1
6	MCP-1	MCP-2	MCP-3	MCSF	MDC	MIG	MIP-1δ	RANTES	SCF	SDF-1	TARC	TGF-ß1
7	TNF-α	TNF-ß	EGF	IGF-1	Angio	Onco	Thrombo	VEGF	PDGF BB	Leptin	Neg	Pos
8	TNF-α	TNF-ß	EGF	IGF-1	Angio	Onco	Thrombo	VEGF	PDGF BB	Leptin	Neg	Pos

Abbreviations: Angio (Angiogenin), Onco (Oncostatin M), Thrombo (Thrombopoietin)

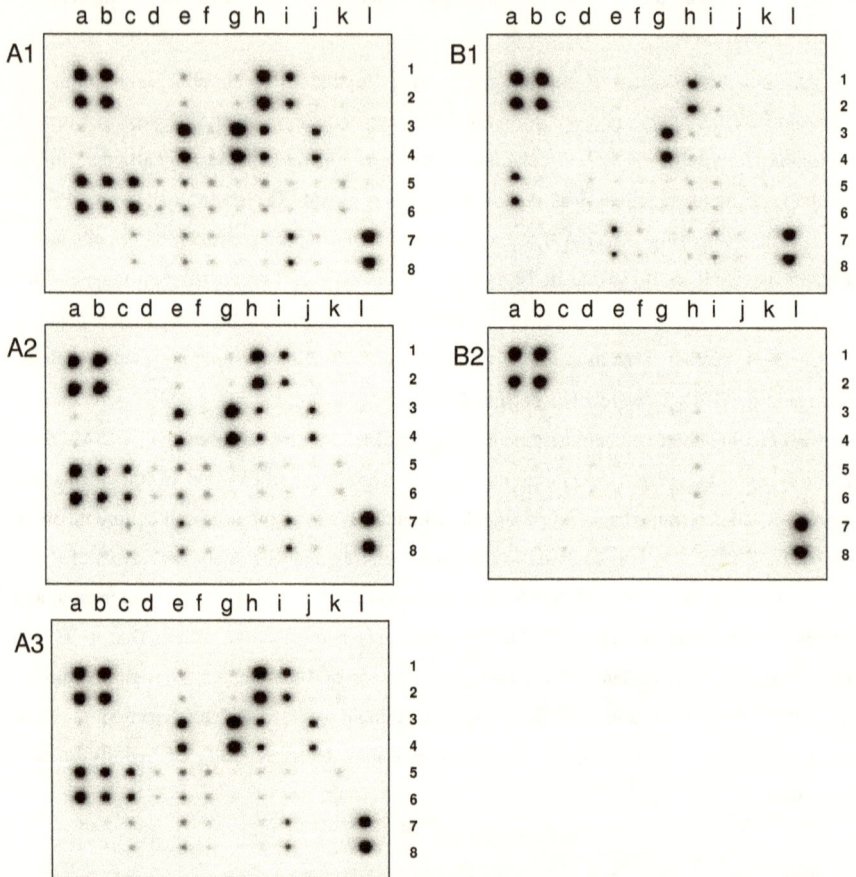

Figure 15. Antiestrogen treatment and altered cytokine secretion in heterologous mixed lymphocyte tumor reactions

MCF-7 cells were seeded in 6-well plates with. After 24 h, treatment with either ethanol (A1), fulvestrant (A2) or 4-hydroxytamoxifen (A3) followed for 2 days. PBMC were applied in a 10:1 ratio for another 4 days. Alternatively, MCF-7 cells were cultivated for 6 days but without application of PBMC (B1). Subsequently, supernatants were collected and cytokine array analyses (Biocat, Heidelberg, Germany) were performed according to the manufacturer´s instructions. To rule out background signals from serum containing medium, DMEM 5% CCS was also assessed (B2).

6.4.5.2 Antiestrogen treatment did not lead to changes in T helper cell differentiation

PBMC were collected from supernatants of heterologous mixed lymphocyte tumor reactions with MCF-7 cells. To determine influences of antiestrogen treatment on the differentiation of Th cells, the subset-specific transcription factors RORγt (Th17 cells), Tbet (Th1 cells) and GATA-3 (Th2 cells) were measured in quantitative real time PCR. As opposed to GATA-3, mRNA expression of RORγt [Fig.16 A] as well as for Tbet [Fig. 16B] was at the detection limit of the real time PCR device. Significant changes in GATA-3 mRNA levels upon antiestrogen treatment of the mixed lymphocyte tumor reaction were not observed [Fig. 16C].

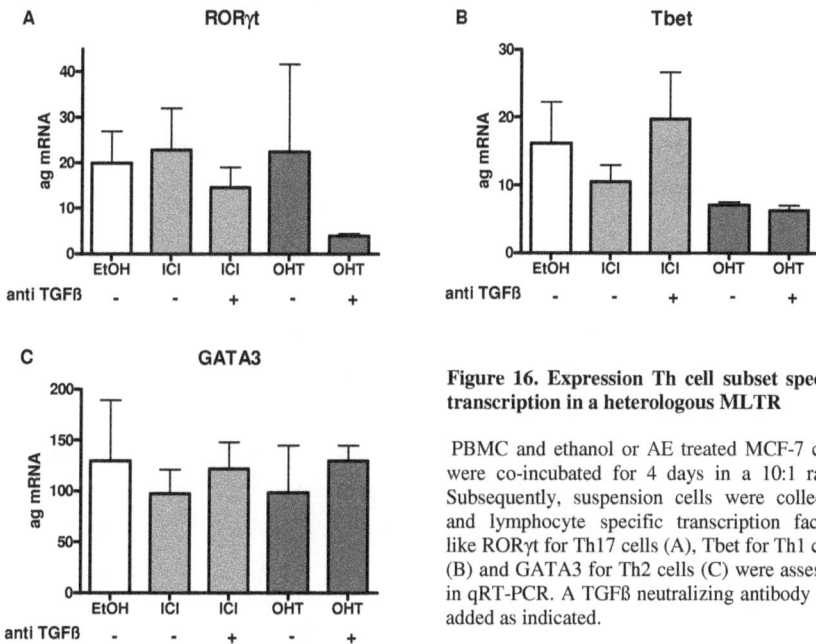

Figure 16. Expression Th cell subset specific transcription in a heterologous MLTR

PBMC and ethanol or AE treated MCF-7 cells were co-incubated for 4 days in a 10:1 ratio. Subsequently, suspension cells were collected and lymphocyte specific transcription factors like RORγt for Th17 cells (A), Tbet for Th1 cells (B) and GATA3 for Th2 cells (C) were assessed in qRT-PCR. A TGFß neutralizing antibody was added as indicated.

73

6.5 Autologous mixed lymphocyte tumor reactions

Among cell culture experiments, approaches with primary cells are most relevant to the actual *in vivo* situation. In the terminal part of this work an autologous mixed lymphocyte tumor reaction was conducted, which means that tumor samples and lymphocytes were obtained from the same individual. In comparison to the usage of cells from varying origins in heterologous mixed lymphocyte tumor reactions, antitumor responses are not artificially enhanced by differences in major histocompatibility complexes. Tumor tissue slices maintaining the original architecture of cancer and stromal cells as well as isolated epithelial tumor cells were used for cytotoxicity assays. Reactivated tumor infiltrating lymphocytes and activated PBMC from the same patient served as effector cells.

6.5.1 Ex vivo AE treatment of primary carcinoma tissue caused induction of Foxp3 expression in autologous TIL

5 large and untreated mammary carcinomas were directly received after surgery and cut into 0.2 mm thick slices with 5 mm in diameter as described by van der Kuip *et al.* (van der Kuip, 2006). The remaining tumor tissue was dissociated for the isolation of EpCAM+ as well as CD3+ cells. After 24 h, tissue slices and tumor cells were treated with ethanol, ICI182.780 or 4-hydroxytamoxifen for 5 days. The isolated CD3+ TIL were reactivated and pooled with PBMC from the same patient to gain a sufficient number of cells for the subsequent autologous MLTR. After 24 hours of coculture with the tumor slices/cells starting on day 4 of antiestrogen treatment, immune cells were collected for RNA isolation. Subsequent qRT-PCR analysis covered lymphocytes in the supernatants as well as CD3+ T cells from within the tissue slices, which were obtained by dissociation. The results provide clear evidence for induction of Foxp3 in lymphocytes isolated from the MLTR with antiestrogen treated tumor slices, which was 3-fold enhanced compared to vehicle treated tumor slices [Fig.17]. Addition of the TGFß neutralizing antibody completely inhibited enhancement of Foxp3 expression. A regulation of cytotoxic effector molecules like GrzmB or perforin was not seen (data not shown).

FoxP3 in TIL

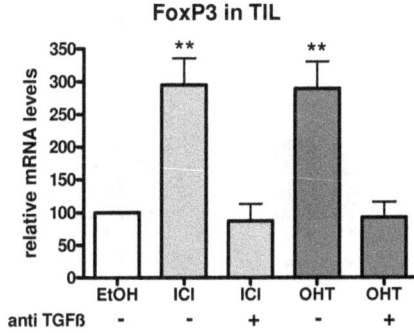

Figure 17. Effect of antiestrogen treatment on the induction of Foxp3 in lymphocytes during an autologous mixed lymphocyte tumor reaction

Tissue slices and EpCAM+ tumor cells were obtained from fresh mammary carcinoma. Both were treated with vehicle, OHT and ICI for 5 days. TILs were also isolated using CD3+ microbeads and reactivated separately with interleukin-2. Autologous PBMC were used to reach sufficient effector cell numbers for the MLTR and activated one day prior to the reaction. After 24 hours of MLTR, suspension cells were harvested and assessed in qRT-PCR. Slices were dissociated to isolate both CD3+ and EpCAM+ cells. Immune cells in suspension and from the slice infiltrate showed similar mRNA expression patterns for Foxp3, with a 3-fold induction when the slices were treated with either OHT or ICI. This effect was reversible with the neutralizing antibody.

6.5.1.1 Antiestrogen treatment did not lead to changes in T helper cell differentiation

PBMC were collected from supernatants of heterologous mixed lymphocyte tumor reactions with MCF-7 cells. To determine influences of antiestrogen treatment on the differentiation of Th cells, the subset-specific transcription factors RORγt (Th17 cells), Tbet (Th1 cells) and GATA-3 (Th2 cells) were measured in quantitative real time PCR. As opposed to GATA-3, mRNA expression of RORγt [Fig.18 A] as well as for Tbet [Fig. 18B] was at the detection limit of the real time PCR device. Significant changes in GATA-3 mRNA levels upon antiestrogen treatment of the mixed lymphocyte tumor reaction were not observed [Fig. 18C].

75

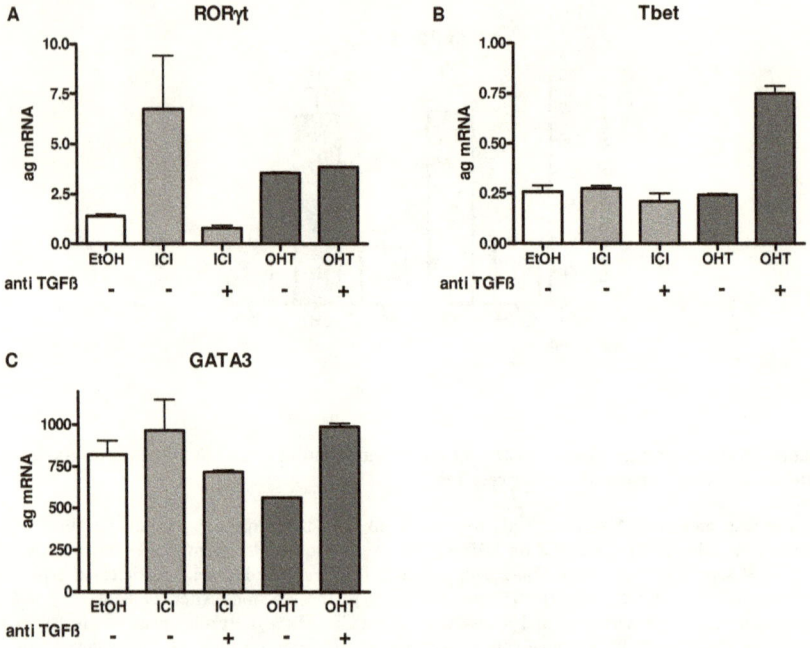

Figure 18. Expression Th cell subset specific transcription factors in an autologous MLTR

Tissue slices and EpCAM+ tumor cells were obtained from fresh mammary carcinoma. Both were treated with vehicle (EtOH), 4-hydroxytamoxifen (OHT) and fulvestrant (ICI) for 5 days. TILs were also isolated using CD3+ microbeads and reactivated separately with interleukin-2. Autologous PBMC were used to reach sufficient effector cell numbers for the MLTR and activated one day prior to the reaction. After 24 hours of MLTR, suspension cells were harvested and assessed in quantitative RT-PCR. Slices were dissociated to isolate both CD3+ and EpCAM+ cells. Immune cells in suspension and from the slice infiltrate showed very low mRNA expression levels for RORγt (A) and Tbet (B). GATA-3 mRNA levels were not significantly regulated by addition of antiestrogens (C).

6.5.2 Quantification of TGFß in tumor slices and supernatants

The CCL64 cell based quantitative TGFß bioassay was used for determination of TGFß in the supernatants of tissue slices and isolated fibroblasts. Conditioned media from slices were collected after the incubation period of 6 days and TGFß was activated via stirring forces. Due to low yield of slices and cells from the tumor samples, this test could only be performed twice. In both cases TGFß concentrations in the supernatants of tumor tissue slices were beyond the sensitivity limit of the assay and exceeded 100 pM even in the ethanol treated controls (data not shown). That points to a high basal secretion level of TGFß as often reported for late stage breast cancer.

6.5.2.1 Quantification of TGFß in supernatants of tumor associated fibroblasts

Tumor associated fibroblasts (TAF) have been reported to increase TGFß production due to tamoxifen treatment. To elucidate their putative participation in antiestrogen induced TGFß secretion in tumors, TAF were isolated and TGFß concentrations in the supernatants after application of antiestrogens were determined. TAF were obtained by cultivation of dissociated tumor tissue cells in cell culture flasks. After removal of EpCAM+ cells by magnetic beads, fibroblasts constitute the cell population, which is prone to adhere on plastic surfaces, whereas TIL can be easily washed away after 1 to 2 days of cultivation. Antiestrogen treatment of fibroblasts for 5 days did not result in increased luciferase activity in cocultured, reporter plasmid transfected CCL64 cells (data not shown).

77

6.5.3 AE treatment reduced the number of apoptotic tumor cells in an autologous MLTR

Aside from the impact on effector cells, target cell apoptosis was assessed in TUNEL assays after antiestrogen treated autologous MLTR. After the reaction, the tissue slices were dissociated and EpCAM+ cells were isolated and fixed on slides for TUNEL staining. Adherent EpCAM+ cells isolated prior to the MLTR were trypsinized and equally processed. In 3 out of 5 cases antiestrogen treatment resulted in a strong decrease of apoptotic, TUNEL positive cells, which was not seen when the TGFß neutralizing antibody was added during the MLTR [Fig.19A, B].

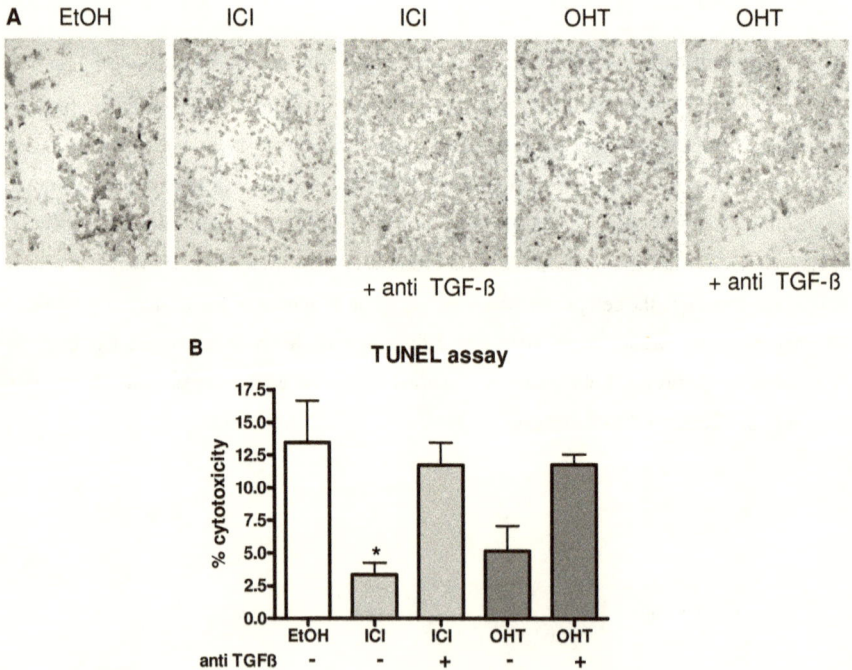

Figure 19. Effect of antiestrogen treatment apoptotic tumor cells in an autologous mixed lymphocyte tumor reaction

The tissue slices were dissociated after 24 hours of mixed lymphocyte tumor reaction and tumor cells were isolated using EpCAM microbeads for subsequent cytospinning. A TUNEL assay was performed to determine the number of apoptotic cells. A) shows a representative set of slides. B) In three out of five cases an AE treatment dependent decrease in TUNEL positive cells was seen. Each cell count was performed by 2 independent investigators.

7 Discussion

Despite the development of new antiestrogen generations and the competing aromatase inhibitors, tamoxifen is still the standard therapy for ER+ breast carcinoma especially in the treatment of pre-menopausal women. Antiestrogens constitute several advantages over other therapeutic regimens, however, resistance to tamoxifen and often concurrently to other, novel antiestrogens frequently arise. Therefore, the elucidation of the underlying mechanisms could help to overcome resistance and thus improve clinical usage of antiestrogens. To gain more insights into antiestrogen induced drug resistance, this study deals with the consequences of TGFß induction in antiestrogen treated breast cancer cells on antitumor immune responses. To address the according questions, cocultures comprising isolated human lymphocyte populations and the hormone responsive mammary carcinoma cell line MCF-7, heterologous mixed lymphocyte and mixed lymphocyte tumor reactions as well as autologous mixed lymphocyte tumor reactions with primary breast cancer cells and reactivated tumor infiltrating lymphocytes were performed.

7.1 Antiestrogens and tumor immunology – a focus on the tumor microenvironment

Clinical data concerning systemic effects of endocrine breast cancer therapy with antiestrogens on the patient´s immune system fail to provide evidence for a noticeable overall immune modulation. Several studies assessed immunological parameters by analyses of peripheral blood from breast cancer patients treated with tamoxifen. Either age-matched groups of patients without hormonal therapy or blood from the monitored patients prior to tamoxifen treatment served as control. In the course of these studies, no altered serum levels of cytokines like interleukin-2, tumor necrosis factor alpha and interferon gamma, which are known to play important roles in antitumor immune responses, could be observed during therapy (Mallmann, 1990 and 1991). Furthermore, no difference in quantity and proportion of several lymphocyte populations like CD4+ T cells, CD8+ T cells and B cells was seen (Mallmann, 1990 and 1991; Sabbioni, 1999). However, conflicting information concerning effects of tamoxifen treatment on natural killer cell quantity and activity derives from the comparison of a work from Berry *et al.* (1987) with studies by Rotstein *et al.* (1988) and Robinson *et al.* (1993). While the former author reports increasing natural killer cell activity in tamoxifen treated patients, Rotstein describes a reduction of their cytotoxicity. This discrepancy is likely to be ascribed to differing lengths of antiestrogen treatment after which natural killer cells function was assessed. Whereas the study by Rotstein *et al.* is based on long term application (1.5 to 2 years), patients in the work of Berry received tamoxifen for only 1 month. The observation that TGFß2 serum levels in tamoxifen responders are elevated (Kopp, 1995) implicates potential effects on peripheral immune cells. However, as already mentioned in the introduction part, TGFß is mainly present in its latent form and requires additional activation steps to fulfil its biological tasks. The lack of constitutive and extensive TGFß activation on a systemic level is likely to be responsible for the absence of an overall immune suppression in patients who respond to tamoxifen and show increased serum levels of TGFß. Nevertheless, systemic blockade of TGFß can augment antitumor responses, which are frequently attenuated by a local immunosuppressive milieu at the tumor site (Kim, 2008). Thus, regarding immunosuppressive effects, antiestrogen induced TGFß production or secretion/activation in cancer cells might primarily be effective in the direct tumor microenvironment.

7.2   Establishment of a MCF-7 cell based coculture with human lymphocytes

To date, the consequences of antiestrogen treatment on the interaction of tumor cells with their immediate surrounding tissue, comprised of stromal fibroblasts, endothelial cells and a variety of infiltrating immune cells are not well understood. A high proportion of the immune cell infiltrate in various cancers is constituted by different lymphocyte subpopulations, which normally hold important functions in the antitumor response. Tumor specific cytotoxic CD8+ T cells can use several mechanisms to directly kill malignant cells, whereas the presence of activated CD4+ T helper cells serves to modulate the antitumor immune response *in situ*. Yet, in many cases tumorigenesis and tumor progression remain largely unaffected despite the presence of effector immune cells. This fact can be due to a lack of cancer specific antigens or to different tumor driven mechanisms including the local production of TGFß. As the expression and secretion/activation of this immunosuppressive growth factor is further induced in breast cancer cells during treatment with antiestrogens (Knabbe, 1987), escape from immune surveillance might be enhanced. To analyze the interaction of antiestrogen treated MCF-7 cells and human CD8+ or CD4+ T lymphocytes, a two chamber system for cocultivation was established. The usage of cell culture inserts with permeable membranes, allowing for exchange of soluble factors, implicates several advantages.

First of all, experiments with conditioned media from antiestrogen treated MCF-7 cells failed to induce luciferase expression in a reporter-gene assay, based on transfection of the TGFß sensitive reporter-plasmid p3TP-lux into mink lung cells (data not shown). This lack of bioactive TGFß seems to be in contradiction to former experiments using p3TP-lux transfected MCF-7 cells for elucidation of autocrine TGFß effects during application of antiestrogens. But it is likely that due to TGFß´s rapid reversion into a latent form during processing of supernatants, no signal can be measured in the subsequent bioassay without further activation steps, e.g. acidic pH. This reasoning was supported by the finding that a direct coculture of p3TP-lux transfected mink lung cells with antiestrogen treated MCF-7 cells resulted in the expected response of the reporter gene assay, as seen by luciferase activity. Therefore, the presence of MCF-7 cells apparently leads to a constant activation of latent TGFß by mechanisms, which were not further investigated in this study. To elucidate direct interactions of the employed breast cancer cell line and human lymphocytes, especially with regard to paracrine effects of TGFß, an insert based coculture seemed most suitable.

Another benefit of this experimental setting derives from the possibility to synchronize activation of T cells and the start of their cocultivation with MCF-7 cells. On the one hand, stimulation of lymphocytes is a precondition for analyses of differential regulation of effector molecules, the expression of which is induced in the course of T cell activation. A widely used *in vitro* activation protocol includes application of both plate-bound CD3 and soluble CD28 antibodies, whereas the former requirement is problematic regarding the MCF-7 pre-cultivation in the cell culture plates. In this context, cell culture inserts can be used as carriers for surface-bound activation antibodies. On the other hand, TGFß is already present in the medium of antiestrogen treated MCF-7 cells when the coculture starts. Its ambiguous effects on lymphocytes are – amongst other things - dependent on the immune cells activation state. Thus, a standardized approach, guaranteeing a robust overall T cell activation and simultaneous impact of tumor cell derived TGFß on the lymphocytes is necessary for inter-experimental comparability.

7.2.1 Inhibition of effector molecule expression in CD8+ cytotoxic T cells

The data from the coculture model fully support the hypothesis that the amount of TGFß produced in a local environment upon induction by antiestrogens suffices to mediate strong inhibition of effector molecule expression in CD8+ T cells. Quantification of secreted and activated TGFß in the reporter gene bioassay highly correlated with results from dose response curves, which served to identify effects of different amounts of TGFß on gene-regulation in

CD8+ T lymphocytes. Western blot analyses confirmed the real time PCR data on effector molecule mRNA transcription in the coculture. In contrast to the constitutive expression and storage of perforin and granzyme protein in human natural killer cells (Fehniger, 2007), granule formation in cytotoxic lymphocytes starts after activation via the T cell receptor (Shresta, 1998). Therefore, inhibiting effects of MCF-7 cell derived TGFß on the effector protein level in lymphocytes could be deteceted after 1 to 2 days and were not distorted by protein amounts already stored in preexisting granules. Several specific antibodies detected recombinant human FasL protein but failed to show FasL in either lysed lymphocytes or – as it is also secreted by CD8+ T cells – in the supernatants of the cocultures. Low FasL protein expression is likely to account for this detection problem. Yet, apart from that, the described findings are in full accordance with recent data from a murine tumor model, in which TGFß was also found to decrease the expression of perforin and granzyme in cytotoxic lymphocytes and where rejection of TGFß secreting EL4 thymoma cells was dependent on neutralization of TGFß activity (Thomas, 2005). As CD8+ cytotoxic effector cells are considered as important players in an antitumor response, their chronic inhibition by TGFß could contribute to tumor evasion from immune surveillance.

7.2.2 Conversion of naïve CD4+ T cells into regulatory T cells

Regulatory T cells (Treg) constitute a further T lymphocyte subset with a central role in tumor immunology, as they can function as suppressors of antitumor responses (Zou, 2006). Three decades ago, Berendt et al. (1980) discovered T cell-mediated suppression of antitumor responses in mice. More recent studies revealed the importance of Foxp3 expression in the development and function of Treg. The cocultivation of naïve CD4+ T cells with antiestrogen treated MCF-7 cells resulted in increased expression of the transcription factor Foxp3, which was completely inhibited by addition of a TGFß neutralizing antibody. Concordantly, Fantini et al. showed inducibility of Foxp3 expression in human CD4+ T cells after in vitro stimulation with TGFß (Fantini, 2004). However, as opposed to Treg differentiation in mice, Foxp3 expression in human CD4+ T cells is not a sufficient condition for the development of suppressive functions. To exclude transient upregulation of Foxp3, which was observed for activated human CD4+ T cells (Allan, 2007), suppressor assays were performed with T cells from the MCF-7 cell cocultures to prove their regulatory function. Continuous stimulation with TGFß was reported to be necessary for maintenance of Treg functions (Selvaraj, 2007). In this context, the assumption that MCF-7 cells provided constant activation of TGFß, which was concluded from lack of TGFß bioactivity in conditioned medium without the presence of MCF-7 cells, might further explain and substantiate the concept of Treg induction in the coculture. Taken together, the CD4+ T cell coculture model suggests that the differentiation and maintenance of functional Foxp3+ Treg in the tumor microenvironment could be enhanced by antiestrogen induced TGFß *in vitro*.

7.3   TGFß effects during the start of an immune response (MLC)

Addition of exogenous interleukin-2, the expression of which is strongly induced upon T cell activation, is known to antagonize TGFß-mediated growth inhibition of lymphocytes (Kehrl, 1986). Given the complex composition of PBMC and the various sources for IL-2 and other cytokines that might overcome TGFß effects during emergence of an (antitumor) immune response, the results from the coculture required further confirmation. As the usage of isolated subpopulations excludes effects, which derive from the interaction of different immune cell subsets, a more integrative approach was realized by performing a mixed lymphocyte culture (MLC). By means of the quantitative bioassay, a relevant TGFß concentration (10 pM) was derived from supernatants of antiestrogen treated MCF-7 cells. The complete inhibition of a MLC typical increase in cell proliferation by application of exogenous TGFß indicated a failure in the development of an immune response. Despite application of rather low doses, a compensation of deleterious TGFß effects on the network of different immune cells can be excluded in this setting and therefore does not seem to be likely during antitumor responses.

7.4   Heterologous mixed lymphocyte tumor reactions

Antiestrogen treatment of MCF-7 cells leads to differential gene regulation in cocultivated lymphocyte subpopulations, which is dependent on the induction of TGFß. As described, this includes the downregulation of effector molecules in CD8+ T cells and induction of Foxp3 in naïve CD4+ lymphocytes, which gave rise to regulatory T cells. Yet, the consequences of these findings on effector cell function during an antitumor response have to be determined. To pursue the results from the coculture system and the mixed lymphocyte reaction, heterologous mixed lymphocyte tumor reactions (MLTR) were performed. Antiestrogen treatment of MCF-7 cells did result in reduced cytotoxicity of PBMC from healthy female donors in a TGFß dependent manner. In general, there are only few studies addressing the direct impact of antiestrogens on the interactions of tumor and immune cells.

A series of works by the group of Berczi *et al.* focused on the hypothesis that patients with estrogen receptor negative cancer like lung carcinoma or mastocytoma might also benefit from antiestrogen treatment (Baral, 1995; Baral, 2000; Nagy, 1997). The application of both tamoxifen and toremifen was used to investigate whether antiestrogens can enhance the immunologic defense of tumor bearing hosts. To this, different cytotoxicity assays were performed with the cell line K562 or with primary cells from human ovarian and lung carcinomas as target. Autologous and heterologous reactions with various effector cells like cytotoxic T lymphocytes (CTL), lymphokine activated killer (LAK) or natural killer cells followed. Pretreatment with antiestrogens significantly enhanced the tumor cell sensitivity to lysis by immune effectors, which, in some cases of ovarian cancer patients, was eventually due to an antiestrogen induced increase in Fas receptor expression (Haeryfar, 2000). Sensitizing effects by pretreatment with tamoxifen or toremifen was also observed in autologous reactions with human lung carcinoma and reactivated tumor infiltrating CTL.

However, these studies rather substantiate than contradict the findings of the work at hand. The induction of TGFß in tumor cells is a prerequisite for the immunosuppression seen in the different approaches of this work. There is evidence that TGFß induction by antiestrogens mainly concerns estrogen receptor positive tumors. The lack of antiestrogen induced enhancement of TGFß expression and secretion/activation in estrogen receptor negative cells was already approved for MDA-MB 231 cells (Knabbe, 1991). As the focus of the present study is on drug resistance mechanisms, which develop during endocrine treatment of estrogen receptor positive mammary carcinomas, two substantially differing systems are investigated. Yet, direct effects of antiestrogens on immune cells remain a critical point.

Despite estrogen receptor independent effects of antiestrogens, their main mode of action appears to be mediated by modulating or inhibiting the receptors transcriptional activity. Thus, expression of one or both isoforms (ERα or ERß) could render immune cells susceptible to antiestrogenic action. Several studies showed ER expression in a variety of cells from the immune system including T and B cells, monocytes and macrophages (Suenaga, 1998; Ben-Hur, 1995). In control experiments of the present work, direct treatment with antiestrogens did not change effector molecule expression in cytotoxic T lymphocytes. Likewise, mRNA levels of the Treg specific transcription factor Foxp3 remained unaffected in CD4+ T cells. Interestingly, physiological levels of estrogens were shown to expand murine Treg cells and to induce expression of Foxp3 in CD4+CD25- T cells, which resulted in the conversion into CD4+CD25+ T cells with suppressive potential (Tai, 2008). However, antagonizing effects of antiestrogens on the TGFß driven differentiation of human Treg cells were not observed in the present study. Despite estrogen depletion by the usage of steroid free serum (CCS) and the presence of 4-hydroxytamoxifen or fulvestrant in the cocultures and in the mixed lymphocyte tumor reactions, functional Treg development occurred. Moreover, at least in the case of tamoxifen, which is referred to as a partial antiestrogen, tissue specific expression of ER cofactors can result in both agonistic and antagonistic action profiles (McDonnell, 1995). While being an antagonist in ER positive breast cancer, a study by Paavonen et al. points to estrogen like effects of tamoxifen in human lymphocytes (Paavonen, 1985), whereas agonizing actions concerning Foxp3 induction were not seen in the present study.

As also shown in the work at hand, pretreatment of PBMC with antiestrogens had no effect on their killing potential in subsequent cytotoxicity assays with untreated MCF-7 cells [Fig. 12A]. This is in accordance with the inability of antiestrogens to directly regulate effector molecules in CD8+ T lypmphocytes. Yet, Drach et al. observed that while mRNA levels of IL-2 in human lymphocytes stayed unaltered during in vitro application of tamoxifen, IL-2 secretion into the extracellular space was strongly reduced (Drach, 1996). Similar results for interferon γ and IL-4 were shown. The authors ascribed these effects to the well-established inhibition of the drug efflux pump P-glycoprotein by tamoxifen. They further concluded that this transport protein has to be involved in secretion of the mentioned cytokines. Several lines of evidence were cited that ruled out P-glycoprotein independent tamoxifen effects on T cell function and activation. Antiestrogen induced retention of mitogenic IL-2, the role of which is central in the activation of cytotoxic effectors like CTL and NK cells during an immune response, might additionally reduce cytotoxicity in tamoxifen treated MLTR. This mechanism could explain the incomplete reversal of reduced cytotoxicity despite neutralization of antiestrogen induced TGFß – an effect that was sometimes observed in the 1 step MLTR. However, comparability to the data in the present work is limited by different amounts of tamoxifen, which was applied in 10- to 50-fold higher concentrations by Drach et al. The lack of systemic changes in IL-2 levels, measured in sera of tamoxifen treated breast cancer patients (Mallmann, 1990, 1991), indicates the complexity of antiestrogenic effects on the immune compartment. This complexity is further accentuated by the finding that IL-2 levels in lymph node cells from tamoxifen treated mice were even increased (Wu, 2000).

As described above, divergent evidence on systemic effects of tamoxifen treatment on NK cell numbers and activity in breast cancer patients exists. Expression of both ERα and ERß has been reported for murine NK cells (Curran, 2001) but a direct impact of antiestrogens on these immune cells has not been elucidated so far. In the present study, antiestrogens strongly inhibited killing of MCF-7 target cells by NK cells from healthy donors via induction of TGFß. This is in full accordance with the finding by Arteaga *et al.* that coadministration of tamoxifen and a neutralizing TGFß antibody overcame tamoxifen resistance of TGFß secreting LCC2 cell tumors in nude mice. As this effect was not observed in beige/nude mice, which lack natural killer cells, the authors concluded immunosuppressive effects of TGFß on NK cells to be central in antiestrogen resistance (Arteaga, 1999). This reasoning is supported by studies showing inhibition of NK cells by TGFß on various levels. This comprised general attenuation of NK cells activity as well as reduced expression of interferon γ, which is essential for stimulation of cell directed Th1 responses (Rook, 1986). Moreover, TGFß signaling in NK cells resulted in downregulation of pattern recognition receptors like NKp30 and NKG2D. As these antigen receptors are needed for activation of NK cells, this leads to a further decrease in cytotoxic activity (Castriconi, 2003).

Participation of TGFß induced regulatory T cells on immunosuppression as demonstrated in this work could also come into play - at least in the 2-step mixed lymphocyte tumor reaction. A 5-day coincubation period in this assay allows for priming of effector lymphocytes, specific for MCF-7 cell antigens. During this time, in which dendritic cells and macrophages are thought to take up and present MCF-7 cell derived peptides to activate specific T cells, Tregs were also induced, as seen by enhanced Foxp3 mRNA levels. Besides direct inhibiting effects of antiestrogen induced TGFß on antigen presenting cells (APC), suppressive T cells could lead to further impairment of the developing antitumor immune response. This includes interference with the APC mediated activation of lymphocytes (Andre, 2009) as well as suppression of CD8+ T and NK cells (Ghiringhelli, 2005; Mempel, 2006).

7.4.1 Cytokine composition and T helper cell differentiation

To investigate the cytokine composition during the heterologous mixed lymphocyte tumor reactions (MLTR) with MCF-7 cells, protein arrays were performed using MLTR supernatants. This approach served to narrow down the influence of cytokines different from TGFß. The mixture of cell signaling molecules like interleukins determines the course of emerging immune responses, mainly by affecting T helper cell differentiation. Several Th subsets can develop, each characterized by a special cytokine expression pattern. The protein arrays revealed the predominance of IL-6, IL-10 and IL-13 during the heterologous MLTR. All of them are referred to as Th2 cytokines. Accordingly, mRNA levels for the Th2 cell specific transcription factor GATA-3 were considerably higher than for T-bet (Th1 cells) and RORγt (Th17 lymphocytes) in

PBMC from the MLTR. However, no differential regulation of GATA-3 mRNA occurred during application of antiestrogens, which is – given the antiestrogen mediated induction of TGFß - in contrast to a study by Gorelik *et al.* (Gorelik, 2000). The authors provide evidence for the inhibition of GATA-3 expression and Th2 cell development by TGFß. The lack of GATA-3 downregulation despite the induction of TGFß by antiestrogens in the MLTR might be explained by dosage effects, whereas the amount Th2 cytokines could outbalance TGFß from MCF-7 cells. The authors applied exogenous TGFß in a 10-fold higher concentration (3 ng/μl) compared to the dosage used in the quantitative bioassay revealed for antiestrogen induced TGFß in MCF-7 cell supernatants in the work at hand (250 pg/μl). In general, the overweight of Th2 cytokines seems to corroborate recent studies on interleukin composition in cancer patients. There are several lines of evidence that a Th2 cell inducing milieu is in favor of tumor progression and tumor evasion from immune surveillance, as it inhibits the development of a cell directed immune response (Lucey, 1996).

As for the mRNA expression of several T cell specific transcription factors, application of antiestrogens during the MLTR did not significantly influence the cytokine composition. A slight reduction in strength of the IL-6, IL-10 and IL-13 signals might derive from TGFß induced overall immunosuppression and its antiproliferative action, implicating less expression and secretion of cytokines. The employed protein array only detects active TGFß. Due to TGFßs rapid reversion into its latent form during processing of supernatants, no signal could be measured. Acid activation of TGFß was not suitable with regard to detection of other cytokines, which do not require activation and may be structurally altered by such a procedure. However, induction of bioactive TGFß in MCF-7 cells upon antiestrogen treatment is well-established (Knabbe, 1987; Knabbe, 1991) and was additionally shown by means of the mink lung cell based TGFß bioassay in the present study [Fig. 3B].

Interestingly, synergistic effects of IL-6 and TGFß were reported to induce Th17 cells during the activation process of CD4+ T cells (Veldhoen, 2006). Of note, both cytokines are present in the MLTR. Nonetheless, a twist in the differentiation of T cells towards a Th17 phenotype did not occur. This was concluded from mRNA expression for the Th17 cell specific transcription factor RORγt, which was at the lower detection limit of the SybrGreen based real time PCR. On the other hand, Treg induction in the MLTR was clearly detectable by enhanced expression of Foxp3 mRNA. Both the development of Th17 cell and Treg requires TGFß, implicating a link in their differentiation. It has been reported that – similar to features of the Th1-Th2 dichotomy – the skewing of T helper cells towards a Treg or a Th17 phenotype in mutually exclusive (Locke, 2009). This correlates with the clear predominance of one of those cell types in the MLTR.

Recent studies concerning the developmental plasticity of Treg and Th17 cells points to a higher flexibility of the latter. Contrarywise, Tregs, once induced by TGFß, are insensitive to Th17 related stimuli like the presence of IL-6 (Zheng, 2008). This could provide an explanation for the induction Treg at the expense of Th17 cells in the MLTR despite the presence of IL-6. TGFß, necessary for the differentiation of both T cell subpopulations, is already present in the MCF-7 cells supernatants when the immune cells are applied. While TGFß is important for the development of induced Treg (Fantini, 2004), its role in Th17 cell differentiation is rather indirect and even dispensable, as reported by Das *et al.* (2009). The authors show that TGFß has no direct effects on the Th17 specific RORγt but instead potentially blocks expression of Th1 and Th2 transcription factors like GATA-3 and signal transducer and activator of transcription (STAT) 4. Moreover, in knockout mice, which are unable to generate Th1 or Th2 cells, TGFß had no effect on Th17 development, whereas IL-6 alone suffices to induce Th17 cells.

7.5 Autologous mixed lymphocyte tumor reactions

The heterologous mixed lymphocyte tumor reaction (MLTR) provided clear evidence for TGFß-mediated immunosuppression during antiestrogen treatment. Yet, the reported data are based on alloreactivity of immune cells against target cells (MCF-7) from another individual. The resulting basal immune reactivity, which is e.g. also seen in host-versus-graft disease, is a consequence of different major histocompatibility complexes (MHC). This mismatch in MHC is unavoidable when cell lines are used in cytotoxicity assays with PBMC and limits the comparability to the *in vivo* situation in breast cancer patients. To substantiate the evidence, which was adduced from the MCF-7 cell based MLTR, reactions with tissue slices from primary mammary carcinoma and autologous immune cells were performed. Only large (> 3 cm) and untreated carcinomas were used in the present study. These inclusion criteria are likely to select for late stage tumors, especially with regard to advanced tumor sizes. Beside the fact that the usage of small, early stage tumors is technically not feasible for the slice model, this focus might implicate several tumor features, which are important for the development of an antiestrogen resistance. The antiproliferative effects of antiestrogens on mammary carcinoma cells are amongst other things due to the induction of the negative growth regulator TGFß (Knabbe, 1987). Its dual role during tumorigenesis implies that late stage tumors frequently become insensitive to TGFß´s inhibitory effects, which might be a meaningful alteration during the development of antiestrogen resistance, too. The initial tumorsuppression by (antiestrogen induced) TGFß can now be turned into cancer promoting effects. Thus, the use of late stage tumors, presumably insensitive to suppressive TGFß action – as supported by high TGFß amounts measured in the slice supernatants – , might better represent a tumor stage in which promoting and paracrine effects of (antiestrogen induced) TGFß are predominant.

To obtain autologous T cells, which are specific for the according tumor antigens, so called tumor infiltrating lymphocytes (TIL) were isolated by means of magnetic anti CD3+ microbeads from the biopsies. These cells were reported to specifically lyse tumor cells after *in vitro* reactivation with IL-2 (Baxevanis, 1994). As sufficient effector cell numbers were scarcely achieved with TIL, autologous PBMC were additionally used in the MLTR with primary breast cancer tissue.

Aside from avoiding artificially enhanced, alloreactive antitumor immunity, the chosen approach, including usage of tissue slices, guaranteed for maintenance of the original tumor architecture. Tumors are composed of heterologous cell types with an intimate interaction profile and provide a rich source for cell signaling molecules that orchestrate tumor progression and/or local immune modulation. Interestingly, fibroblasts, which are frequently found to reside in solid tumors, were reported to enhance secretion of TGFß upon antiestrogen application *in vitro* (Colletta, 1990) and *in vivo* (Butta, 1992). However, none of the fibroblasts isolated from breast cancer biopsies in the present study showed increased TGFß release during treatment with tamoxifen or fulvestrant, as determined by the TGFß bioassay (data not shown).

In 3 cases, in which quantification of TGFß from the tumor slice supernatants was performed, the analysis was complicated by TGFß amounts that exceeded the upper detection limit of the bioassay. Yet, a release of 100-400 pM TGFß could be extrapolated. The high basal secretion of the used late stage tumors might account for differences in lymphocyte effector molecule expression concerning the heterologous versus the autologous MLTR. In contrast to the induction of Foxp3 in the autologous MLTR, no further downregulation of lymphocyte effector molecules like GzmB or perforin was observed when antiestrogens were applied. Dose response curves demonstrated that GzmB and perforin downregulation was highly TGFß sensitive, with small amounts (10-30 pM) resulting in an early plateau of inhibition, as opposed to the induction of Foxp3 displaying a different dose response profile with further increases at higher TGFß doses. Nevertheless, TUNEL staining showed that antiestrogen treatment in the autologous MLTR led to less apoptotic tumor cells in 3 out of 5 cases analyzed. Of note, in all cases where antiestrogens affected tumor cell apoptosis, addition of a neutralizing TGFß antibody reversed this action. A direct inhibition of apoptosis by TGFß could be ruled out for doxorubicin treated MCF-7 cells and therefore appears to be unlikely also for primary tumor cells.

The increase of Foxp3 in the autologous MLTR is in accordance with the hypothesis that the tumor driven accumulation or generation of Treg and the resulting local immune tolerance can be responsible for further tumor progression (Bohling, 2008). Mechanistically, once activated by the tumor cell derived TGFß, Tregs can interfere with the activation and differentiation of naïve T cells towards mounting a cytotoxic effector cell response. For example, high expression of the IL-2 receptor α chain (CD25) on Tregs could lead to a competitive binding of IL-2, thereby depriving naïve lymphocytes from expansion and differentiation signals into effector T cells (Vignali, 2008). In addition, expression of soluble or membrane-bound immunosuppressive factors like TGFß or interleukin-10 by Treg can further attenuate tumor specific responses through direct interference with cytotoxic effector cell function of both NK and CTL. Furthermore, recent studies revealed that Treg are able to suppress or kill antigen presenting cells (APC), too, substantially widening the field of Treg action (Andre, 2009). The inhibition of APC function by Treg can be mediated via TGFß, which has been shown to compromise antigen presentation on dendritic cells or macrophages, e.g. by downregulation of T cell co-stimulatory molecules or MHCII (Brown, 2001; Lee, 1997). Treg mediated impairment of APC functions in turn can lead to an early abrogation of T cell activation already during the priming process. Thus, the reduced number of apoptotic tumor cells observed in the autologous MLTR is likely to originate largely from the antiestrogen induced, TGFß-mediated induction of Foxp3 positive Tregs within the lymphocytes, which may become effective at various levels of activation of a tumor specific cytotoxic effector cell response. Although not assessed in this study, in addition to the TGFß-mediated inhibition of APCs, a concomitant direct antiestrogen mediated interference with dendritic cell differentiation, as previously reported (Nalbandian, 2005), may further contribute to tumor escape from immune surveillance (Kusmartsev, 2006).

7.6 Conclusions and outlook

Heterologous and autologous mixed lymphocyte tumor reactions clearly showed reduced cytotoxicity of immune effector cells when tumor target cells were treated with 4-hydroxytamoxifen or fulvestrant. In the former case TGFß dependent downregulation of effector molecules in CTL and induction of regulatory T cells account for less killing potential. In the autologous MLTR inhibition of CTL was not further augmented by antiestrogen induced TGFß, which on the other hand led to induction of Foxp3 positive T cells. Determination of apoptotic tumor cells from autologous MLTR indicated less killing during antitumor responses when antiestrogens were applied. All effects were reversible by addition of a TGFß neutralizing antibody.

Taken together, the present data are pointing at a putative drug resistance mechanism, by which antiestrogen treatment may help tumor cells to evade from immune surveillance through the induction of TGFß. The research field of tumor immunology is constantly advancing but the link between antiestrogen therapy of ER+ breast cancer and the potential causation of immune modulation has not gained much attention. Nevertheless, emergence or enhancement of TGFß driven immunosuppression during application of antiestrogens could critically contribute to the development of drug resistance. To overcome these tumor promoting side effects, cotreatment with TGFß antagonizing compounds could be considered. Yet, this approach should be assessed with caution, as the effects of (antiestrogen induced) TGFß on cancer depend on both the tumor stage and its individual constitution. Inhibiting, autocrine TGFß effects, which are desirable, could also be prevented by antagonists. Another solution could be the concomitant stimulation of the antitumor response, as aimed for in the multifaceted approaches that are used in immunotherapy of cancer. This includes vaccination strategies, adoptive transfer of *ex vivo* stimulated immune cells and usage of bispecific antibodies, which can recruit and activate cytotoxic T cells.

8 Reference List

(1) Ahamed J, Burg N, Yoshinaga K, Janczak CA, Rifkin DB, Coller BS. In vitro and in vivo evidence for shear-induced activation of latent transforming growth factor-beta1. Blood 2008 Nov 1;112(9):3650-60.

(2) Allan SE, Crome SQ, Crellin NK, Passerini L, Steiner TS, Bacchetta R, et al. Activation-induced FOXP3 in human T effector cells does not suppress proliferation or cytokine production. Int Immunol 2007 Apr;19(4):345-54.

(3) Andre S, Tough DF, Lacroix-Desmazes S, Kaveri SV, Bayry J. Surveillance of antigen-presenting cells by CD4+ CD25+ regulatory T cells in autoimmunity: immunopathogenesis and therapeutic implications. Am J Pathol 2009 May;174(5):1575-87.

(4) Annes JP, Munger JS, Rifkin DB. Making sense of latent TGFbeta activation. J Cell Sci 2003 Jan 15;116(Pt 2):217-24.

(5) Arpino G, Wiechmann L, Osborne CK, Schiff R. Crosstalk between the estrogen receptor and the HER tyrosine kinase receptor family: molecular mechanism and clinical implications for endocrine therapy resistance. Endocr Rev 2008 Apr;29(2):217-33.

(6) Arteaga CL, Koli KM, Dugger TC, Clarke R. Reversal of tamoxifen resistance of human breast carcinomas in vivo by neutralizing antibodies to transforming growth factor-beta. J Natl Cancer Inst 1999 Jan 6;91(1):46-53.

(7) Baral E, Nagy E, Berczi I. Modulation of natural killer cell-mediated cytotoxicity by tamoxifen and estradiol. Cancer 1995 Jan 15;75(2):591-9.

(8) Baral E, Nagy E, Krepart GV, Lotocki RJ, Unruh HW, Berczi I. Antiestrogens sensitize human ovarian and lung carcinomas for lysis by autologous killer cells. Anticancer Res 2000 May;20(3B):2027-31.

(9) Barcellos-Hoff MH, Derynck R, Tsang ML, Weatherbee JA. Transforming growth factor-beta activation in irradiated murine mammary gland. J Clin Invest 1994

Feb;93(2):892-9.

(10) Barry M, Bleackley RC. Cytotoxic T lymphocytes: all roads lead to death. Nat Rev Immunol 2002 Jun;2(6):401-9.

(11) Bates GJ, Fox SB, Han C, Leek RD, Garcia JF, Harris AL, et al. Quantification of regulatory T cells enables the identification of high-risk breast cancer patients and those at risk of late relapse. J Clin Oncol 2006 Dec 1;24(34):5373-80.

(12) Baxevanis CN, Dedoussis GV, Papadopoulos NG, Missitzis I, Stathopoulos GP, Papamichail M. Tumor specific cytolysis by tumor infiltrating lymphocytes in breast cancer. Cancer 1994 Aug 15;74(4):1275-82.

(13) Beisner J, Buck MB, Fritz P, Dippon J, Schwab M, Brauch H, et al. A novel functional polymorphism in the transforming growth factor-beta2 gene promoter and tumor progression in breast cancer. Cancer Res 2006 Aug 1;66(15):7554-61.

(14) Ben-Hur H, Mor G, Insler V, Blickstein I, mir-Zaltsman Y, Sharp A, et al. Menopause is associated with a significant increase in blood monocyte number and a relative decrease in the expression of estrogen receptors in human peripheral monocytes. Am J Reprod Immunol 1995 Dec;34(6):363-9.

(15) Berendt MJ, North RJ. T-cell-mediated suppression of anti-tumor immunity. An explanation for progressive growth of an immunogenic tumor. J Exp Med 1980 Jan 1;151(1):69-80.

(16) Berry J, Green BJ, Matheson DS. Modulation of natural killer cell activity by tamoxifen in stage I post-menopausal breast cancer. Eur J Cancer Clin Oncol 1987 May;23(5):517-20.

(17) Bogdan C, Paik J, Vodovotz Y, Nathan C. Contrasting mechanisms for suppression of macrophage cytokine release by transforming growth factor-beta and interleukin-10. J Biol Chem 1992 Nov 15;267(32):23301-8.

(18) Bohling SD, Allison KH. Immunosuppressive regulatory T cells are associated with aggressive breast cancer phenotypes: a potential therapeutic target. Mod Pathol 2008 Dec;21(12):1527-32.

(19) Brown RD, Pope B, Murray A, Esdale W, Sze DM, Gibson J, et al. Dendritic cells from patients with myeloma are numerically normal but functionally defective as they fail to up-regulate CD80 (B7-1) expression after huCD40LT stimulation because of inhibition by transforming growth factor-beta1 and interleukin-10. Blood 2001 Nov 15;98(10):2992-8.

(20) Butta A, MacLennan K, Flanders KC, Sacks NP, Smith I, McKinna A, et al. Induction of transforming growth factor beta 1 in human breast cancer in vivo following tamoxifen treatment. Cancer Res 1992 Aug 1;52(15):4261-4.

(21) Byrne SN, Knox MC, Halliday GM. TGFbeta is responsible for skin tumour infiltration by macrophages enabling the tumours to escape immune destruction. Immunol Cell Biol 2008 Jan;86(1):92-7.

(22) Cao X, Cai SF, Fehniger TA, Song J, Collins LI, Piwnica-Worms DR, et al. Granzyme B and perforin are important for regulatory T cell-mediated suppression of tumor clearance. Immunity 2007 Oct;27(4):635-46.

(23) Castriconi R, Cantoni C, Della CM, Vitale M, Marcenaro E, Conte R, et al. Transforming growth factor beta 1 inhibits expression of NKp30 and NKG2D receptors: consequences for the NK-mediated killing of dendritic cells. Proc Natl Acad Sci U S A 2003 Apr 1;100(7):4120-5.

(24) Cederbom L, Hall H, Ivars F. CD4+CD25+ regulatory T cells down-regulate co-stimulatory molecules on antigen-presenting cells. Eur J Immunol 2000 Jun;30(6):1538-43.

(25) Chen CH, Seguin-Devaux C, Burke NA, Oriss TB, Watkins SC, Clipstone N, et al. Transforming growth factor beta blocks Tec kinase phosphorylation, Ca2+ influx, and NFATc translocation causing inhibition of T cell differentiation. J Exp Med 2003 Jun 16;197(12):1689-99.

(26) Colletta AA, Wakefield LM, Howell FV, van Roozendaal KE, Danielpour D, Ebbs SR, et al. Anti-oestrogens induce the secretion of active transforming growth factor beta from human fetal fibroblasts. Br J Cancer 1990 Sep;62(3):405-9.

(27) Condeelis J, Pollard JW. Macrophages: obligate partners for tumor cell migration,

invasion, and metastasis. Cell 2006 Jan 27;124(2):263-6.

(28) Curran EM, Berghaus LJ, Vernetti NJ, Saporita AJ, Lubahn DB, Estes DM. Natural killer cells express estrogen receptor-alpha and estrogen receptor-beta and can respond to estrogen via a non-estrogen receptor-alpha-mediated pathway. Cell Immunol 2001 Nov 25;214(1):12-20.

(29) Das J, Ren G, Zhang L, Roberts AI, Zhao X, Bothwell AL, et al. Transforming growth factor beta is dispensable for the molecular orchestration of Th17 cell differentiation. J Exp Med 2009 Oct 26;206(11):2407-16.

(30) de Jong JS, van Diest PJ, van d, V, Baak JP. Expression of growth factors, growth-inhibiting factors, and their receptors in invasive breast cancer. II: Correlations with proliferation and angiogenesis. J Pathol 1998 Jan;184(1):53-7.

(31) Derynck R, Akhurst RJ, Balmain A. TGF-beta signaling in tumor suppression and cancer progression. Nat Genet 2001 Oct;29(2):117-29.

(32) Drach J, Gsur A, Hamilton G, Zhao S, Angerler J, Fiegl M, et al. Involvement of P-glycoprotein in the transmembrane transport of interleukin-2 (IL-2), IL-4, and interferon-gamma in normal human T lymphocytes. Blood 1996 Sep 1;88(5):1747-54.

(33) Emery J, Lucassen A, Murphy M. Common hereditary cancers and implications for primary care. Lancet 2001 Jul 7;358(9275):56-63.

(34) Engle SJ, Hoying JB, Boivin GP, Ormsby I, Gartside PS, Doetschman T. Transforming growth factor beta1 suppresses nonmetastatic colon cancer at an early stage of tumorigenesis. Cancer Res 1999 Jul 15;59(14):3379-86.

(35) Fantini MC, Becker C, Monteleone G, Pallone F, Galle PR, Neurath MF. Cutting edge: TGF-beta induces a regulatory phenotype in CD4+. J Immunol 2004 May 1;172(9):5149-53.

(36) Fehniger TA, Cai SF, Cao X, Bredemeyer AJ, Presti RM, French AR, et al. Acquisition of murine NK cell cytotoxicity requires the translation of a pre-existing pool of granzyme B and perforin mRNAs. Immunity 2007 Jun;26(6):798-811.

(37) Forrester E, Chytil A, Bierie B, Aakre M, Gorska AE, Sharif-Afshar AR, et al. Effect of

95

conditional knockout of the type II TGF-beta receptor gene in mammary epithelia on mammary gland development and polyomavirus middle T antigen induced tumor formation and metastasis. Cancer Res 2005 Mar 15;65(6):2296-302.

(38) Friedman E, Gold LI, Klimstra D, Zeng ZS, Winawer S, Cohen A. High levels of transforming growth factor beta 1 correlate with disease progression in human colon cancer. Cancer Epidemiol Biomarkers Prev 1995 Jul;4(5):549-54.

(39) Gajdusek CM, Luo Z, Mayberg MR. Basic fibroblast growth factor and transforming growth factor beta-1: synergistic mediators of angiogenesis in vitro. J Cell Physiol 1993 Oct;157(1):133-44.

(40) Geissmann F, Revy P, Regnault A, Lepelletier Y, Dy M, Brousse N, et al. TGF-beta 1 prevents the noncognate maturation of human dendritic Langerhans cells. J Immunol 1999 Apr 15;162(8):4567-75.

(41) Gershon RK. A disquisition on suppressor T cells. Transplant Rev 1975;26:170-85.

(42) Ghiringhelli F, Menard C, Terme M, Flament C, Taieb J, Chaput N, et al. CD4+CD25+ regulatory T cells inhibit natural killer cell functions in a transforming factor-beta-dependent manner. J Exp Med 2005 Oct 17;202(8):1075-85.

(43) Ghiringhelli F, Menard C, Martin F, Zitvogel L. The role of regulatory T cells in the control of natural killer cells: relevance during tumor progression. Immunol Rev 2006 Dec;214:229-38.

(44) Glick AB, Weinberg WC, Wu IH, Quan W, Yuspa SH. Transforming growth factor beta 1 suppresses genomic instability independent of a G1 arrest, p53, and Rb. Cancer Res 1996 Aug 15;56(16):3645-50.

(45) Gobbi H, Arteaga CL, Jensen RA, Simpson JF, Dupont WD, Olson SJ, et al. Loss of expression of transforming growth factor beta type II receptor correlates with high tumour grade in human breast in-situ and invasive carcinomas. Histopathology 2000 Feb;36(2):168-77.

(46) Gold LI. The role for transforming growth factor-beta (TGF-beta) in human cancer. Crit Rev Oncog 1999;10(4):303-60.

(47) Gorelik L, Flavell RA. Abrogation of TGFbeta signaling in T cells leads to spontaneous T cell differentiation and autoimmune disease. Immunity 2000 Feb;12(2):171-81.

(48) Gorelik L, Fields PE, Flavell RA. Cutting edge: TGF-beta inhibits Th type 2 development through inhibition of GATA-3 expression. J Immunol 2000 Nov 1;165(9):4773-7.

(49) Gorelik L, Flavell RA. Immune-mediated eradication of tumors through the blockade of transforming growth factor-beta signaling in T cells. Nat Med 2001 Oct;7(10):1118-22.

(50) Gorska AE, Jensen RA, Shyr Y, Aakre ME, Bhowmick NA, Moses HL. Transgenic mice expressing a dominant-negative mutant type II transforming growth factor-beta receptor exhibit impaired mammary development and enhanced mammary tumor formation. Am J Pathol 2003 Oct;163(4):1539-49.

(51) Gutierrez MC, Detre S, Johnston S, Mohsin SK, Shou J, Allred DC, et al. Molecular changes in tamoxifen-resistant breast cancer: relationship between estrogen receptor, HER-2, and p38 mitogen-activated protein kinase. J Clin Oncol 2005 Apr 10;23(11):2469-76.

(52) Haeryfar SM, Nagy E, Baral E, Krepart G, Lotocki R, Berczi I. Antiestrogens affect both pathways of killer cell-mediated oncolysis. Anticancer Res 2000 May;20(3A):1849-53.

(53) Han J, Hajjar DP, Tauras JM, Feng J, Gotto AM, Jr., Nicholson AC. Transforming growth factor-beta1 (TGF-beta1) and TGF-beta2 decrease expression of CD36, the type B scavenger receptor, through mitogen-activated protein kinase phosphorylation of peroxisome proliferator-activated receptor-gamma. J Biol Chem 2000 Jan 14;275(2):1241-6.

(54) Harrington LE, Hatton RD, Mangan PR, Turner H, Murphy TL, Murphy KM, et al. Interleukin 17-producing CD4+ effector T cells develop via a lineage distinct from the T helper type 1 and 2 lineages. Nat Immunol 2005 Nov;6(11):1123-32.

(55) Harvey JM, Clark GM, Osborne CK, Allred DC. Estrogen receptor status by immunohistochemistry is superior to the ligand-binding assay for predicting response to

adjuvant endocrine therapy in breast cancer. J Clin Oncol 1999 May;17(5):1474-81.

(56) Huber MA, Kraut N, Beug H. Molecular requirements for epithelial-mesenchymal transition during tumor progression. Curr Opin Cell Biol 2005 Oct;17(5):548-58.

(57) Jordan VC. Fourteenth Gaddum Memorial Lecture. A current view of tamoxifen for the treatment and prevention of breast cancer. Br J Pharmacol 1993 Oct;110(2):507-17.

(58) Kehrl JH, Wakefield LM, Roberts AB, Jakowlew S, varez-Mon M, Derynck R, et al. Production of transforming growth factor beta by human T lymphocytes and its potential role in the regulation of T cell growth. J Exp Med 1986 May 1;163(5):1037-50.

(59) Khattri R, Kasprowicz D, Cox T, Mortrud M, Appleby MW, Brunkow ME, et al. The amount of scurfin protein determines peripheral T cell number and responsiveness. J Immunol 2001 Dec 1;167(11):6312-20.

(60) Kim S, Buchlis G, Fridlender ZG, Sun J, Kapoor V, Cheng G, et al. Systemic blockade of transforming growth factor-beta signaling augments the efficacy of immunogene therapy. Cancer Res 2008 Dec 15;68(24):10247-56.

(61) Kim SJ, Im YH, Markowitz SD, Bang YJ. Molecular mechanisms of inactivation of TGF-beta receptors during carcinogenesis. Cytokine Growth Factor Rev 2000 Mar;11(1-2):159-68.

(62) Kim YJ, Stringfield TM, Chen Y, Broxmeyer HE. Modulation of cord blood CD8+ T-cell effector differentiation by TGF-beta1 and 4-1BB costimulation. Blood 2005 Jan 1;105(1):274-81.

(63) Klinge CM. Estrogen receptor interaction with estrogen response elements. Nucleic Acids Res 2001 Jul 15;29(14):2905-19.

(64) Knabbe C, Lippman ME, Wakefield LM, Flanders KC, Kasid A, Derynck R, et al. Evidence that transforming growth factor-beta is a hormonally regulated negative growth factor in human breast cancer cells. Cell 1987 Feb 13;48(3):417-28.

(65) Knabbe C, Zugmaier G, Schmahl M, Dietel M, Lippman ME, Dickson RB. Induction of transforming growth factor beta by the antiestrogens droloxifene, tamoxifen, and

toremifene in MCF-7 cells. Am J Clin Oncol 1991;14 Suppl 2:S15-S20.

(66) Knabbe C, Kopp A, Hilgers W, Lang D, Muller V, Zugmaier G, et al. Regulation and role of TGF beta production in breast cancer. Ann N Y Acad Sci 1996 Apr 30;784:263-76.

(67) Kopp A, Jonat W, Schmahl M, Knabbe C. Transforming growth factor beta 2 (TGF-beta 2) levels in plasma of patients with metastatic breast cancer treated with tamoxifen. Cancer Res 1995 Oct 15;55(20):4512-5.

(68) Kopp HG, Placke T, Salih HR. Platelet-derived transforming growth factor-beta down-regulates NKG2D thereby inhibiting natural killer cell antitumor reactivity. Cancer Res 2009 Oct 1;69(19):7775-83.

(69) Kumar R, Kamdar D, Madden L, Hills C, Crooks D, O'Brien D, et al. Th1/Th2 cytokine imbalance in meningioma, anaplastic astrocytoma and glioblastoma multiforme patients. Oncol Rep 2006 Jun;15(6):1513-6.

(70) Kusmartsev S, Gabrilovich DI. Effect of tumor-derived cytokines and growth factors on differentiation and immune suppressive features of myeloid cells in cancer. Cancer Metastasis Rev 2006 Sep;25(3):323-31.

(71) Lee YJ, Han Y, Lu HT, Nguyen V, Qin H, Howe PH, et al. TGF-beta suppresses IFN-gamma induction of class II MHC gene expression by inhibiting class II transactivator messenger RNA expression. J Immunol 1997 Mar 1;158(5):2065-75.

(72) Li MO, Sanjabi S, Flavell RA. Transforming growth factor-beta controls development, homeostasis, and tolerance of T cells by regulatory T cell-dependent and -independent mechanisms. Immunity 2006 Sep;25(3):455-71.

(73) Li MO, Wan YY, Sanjabi S, Robertson AK, Flavell RA. Transforming growth factor-beta regulation of immune responses. Annu Rev Immunol 2006;24:99-146.

(74) Li MO, Flavell RA. TGF-beta: a master of all T cell trades. Cell 2008 Aug 8;134(3):392-404.

(75) Lippman ME, Dickson RB, Gelmann EP, Rosen N, Knabbe C, Bates S, et al. Growth regulatory peptide production by human breast carcinoma cells. J Steroid Biochem

1988;30(1-6):53-61.

(76) Lo RS, Wotton D, Massague J. Epidermal growth factor signaling via Ras controls the Smad transcriptional co-repressor TGIF. EMBO J 2001 Jan 15;20(1-2):128-36.

(77) Locke NR, Patterson SJ, Hamilton MJ, Sly LM, Krystal G, Levings MK. SHIP regulates the reciprocal development of T regulatory and Th17 cells. J Immunol 2009 Jul 15;183(2):975-83.

(78) Lucey DR, Clerici M, Shearer GM. Type 1 and type 2 cytokine dysregulation in human infectious, neoplastic, and inflammatory diseases. Clin Microbiol Rev 1996 Oct;9(4):532-62.

(79) Ludviksson BR, Seegers D, Resnick AS, Strober W. The effect of TGF-beta1 on immune responses of naive versus memory CD4+ Th1/Th2 T cells. Eur J Immunol 2000 Jul;30(7):2101-11.

(80) Lyon MF, Peters J, Glenister PH, Ball S, Wright E. The scurfy mouse mutant has previously unrecognized hematological abnormalities and resembles Wiskott-Aldrich syndrome. Proc Natl Acad Sci U S A 1990 Apr;87(7):2433-7.

(81) Lyons RM, Keski-Oja J, Moses HL. Proteolytic activation of latent transforming growth factor-beta from fibroblast-conditioned medium. J Cell Biol 1988 May;106(5):1659-65.

(82) Ma A, Koka R, Burkett P. Diverse functions of IL-2, IL-15, and IL-7 in lymphoid homeostasis. Annu Rev Immunol 2006;24:657-79.

(83) MacCallum J, Keen JC, Bartlett JM, Thompson AM, Dixon JM, Miller WR. Changes in expression of transforming growth factor beta mRNA isoforms in patients undergoing tamoxifen therapy. Br J Cancer 1996 Aug;74(3):474-8.

(84) Maehara Y, Kakeji Y, Kabashima A, Emi Y, Watanabe A, Akazawa K, et al. Role of transforming growth factor-beta 1 in invasion and metastasis in gastric carcinoma. J Clin Oncol 1999 Feb;17(2):607-14.

(85) Mallmann P, Dietrich K, Krebs D. Effect of tamoxifen and high-dose medroxyprogesterone acetate (MPA) on cell-mediated immune functions in breast

cancer patients. Methods Find Exp Clin Pharmacol 1990 Dec;12(10):699-706.

(86) Mallmann P, Krebs D. [Effect of tamoxifen on parameters of cell-mediated immunity in postmenopausal patients with breast carcinoma]. Zentralbl Gynakol 1991;113(12):689-96.

(87) Massague J. TGFbeta in Cancer. Cell 2008 Jul 25;134(2):215-30.

(88) McDonnell DP, Clemm DL, Hermann T, Goldman ME, Pike JW. Analysis of estrogen receptor function in vitro reveals three distinct classes of antiestrogens. Mol Endocrinol 1995 Jun;9(6):659-69.

(89) Mempel TR, Pittet MJ, Khazaie K, Weninger W, Weissleder R, von BH, et al. Regulatory T cells reversibly suppress cytotoxic T cell function independent of effector differentiation. Immunity 2006 Jul;25(1):129-41.

(90) Nagy E, Baral E, Kangas L, Berczi I. Anti-estrogens potentiate the immunotherapy of the P815 murine mastocytoma by cytotoxic T lymphocytes. Anticancer Res 1997 Mar;17(2A):1083-8.

(91) Nalbandian G, Paharkova-Vatchkova V, Mao A, Nale S, Kovats S. The selective estrogen receptor modulators, tamoxifen and raloxifene, impair dendritic cell differentiation and activation. J Immunol 2005 Aug 15;175(4):2666-75.

(92) Nilsson S, Makela S, Treuter E, Tujague M, Thomsen J, Andersson G, et al. Mechanisms of estrogen action. Physiol Rev 2001 Oct;81(4):1535-65.

(93) Nishikawa H, Kato T, Tawara I, Takemitsu T, Saito K, Wang L, et al. Accelerated chemically induced tumor development mediated by CD4+CD25+ regulatory T cells in wild-type hosts. Proc Natl Acad Sci U S A 2005 Jun 28;102(26):9253-7.

(94) O'Garra A. Cytokines induce the development of functionally heterogeneous T helper cell subsets. Immunity 1998 Mar;8(3):275-83.

(95) Ormandy LA, Hillemann T, Wedemeyer H, Manns MP, Greten TF, Korangy F. Increased populations of regulatory T cells in peripheral blood of patients with hepatocellular carcinoma. Cancer Res 2005 Mar 15;65(6):2457-64.

(96) Osborne CK, Arteaga CL. Autocrine and paracrine growth regulation of breast cancer:

clinical implications. Breast Cancer Res Treat 1990 Jan;15(1):3-11.

(97) Paavonen T, Andersson LC. The oestrogen antagonists, tamoxifen and FC-1157a, display oestrogen like effects on human lymphocyte functions in vitro. Clin Exp Immunol 1985 Aug;61(2):467-74.

(98) Padua D, Massague J. Roles of TGFbeta in metastasis. Cell Res 2009 Jan;19(1):89-102.

(99) Peng Y, Laouar Y, Li MO, Green EA, Flavell RA. TGF-beta regulates in vivo expansion of Foxp3-expressing CD4+CD25+ regulatory T cells responsible for protection against diabetes. Proc Natl Acad Sci U S A 2004 Mar 30;101(13):4572-7.

(100) Petrocca F, Visone R, Onelli MR, Shah MH, Nicoloso MS, de M, I, et al. E2F1-regulated microRNAs impair TGFbeta-dependent cell-cycle arrest and apoptosis in gastric cancer. Cancer Cell 2008 Mar;13(3):272-86.

(101) Pierce DF, Jr., Gorska AE, Chytil A, Meise KS, Page DL, Coffey RJ, Jr., et al. Mammary tumor suppression by transforming growth factor beta 1 transgene expression. Proc Natl Acad Sci U S A 1995 May 9;92(10):4254-8.

(102) Rachez C, Freedman LP. Mediator complexes and transcription. Curr Opin Cell Biol 2001 Jun;13(3):274-80.

(103) Roberts AB, Sporn MB, Assoian RK, Smith JM, Roche NS, Wakefield LM, et al. Transforming growth factor type beta: rapid induction of fibrosis and angiogenesis in vivo and stimulation of collagen formation in vitro. Proc Natl Acad Sci U S A 1986 Jun;83(12):4167-71.

(104) Robinson E, Rubin D, Mekori T, Segal R, Pollack S. In vivo modulation of natural killer cell activity by tamoxifen in patients with bilateral primary breast cancer. Cancer Immunol Immunother 1993 Aug;37(3):209-12.

(105) Roodi N, Bailey LR, Kao WY, Verrier CS, Yee CJ, Dupont WD, et al. Estrogen receptor gene analysis in estrogen receptor-positive and receptor-negative primary breast cancer. J Natl Cancer Inst 1995 Mar 15;87(6):446-51.

(106) Rook AH, Kehrl JH, Wakefield LM, Roberts AB, Sporn MB, Burlington DB, et al. Effects of transforming growth factor beta on the functions of natural killer cells:

depressed cytolytic activity and blunting of interferon responsiveness. J Immunol 1986 May 15;136(10):3916-20.

(107) Rotstein S, Blomgren H, Petrini B, Wasserman J, von Stedingk LV. Influence of adjuvant tamoxifen on blood lymphocytes. Breast Cancer Res Treat 1988 Sep;12(1):75-9.

(108) Sabbioni ME, Castiglione M, Hurny C, Siegrist HP, Bacchi M, Bernhard J, et al. Interaction of tamoxifen with concurrent cytotoxic adjuvant treatment affects lymphocytes and lymphocyte subsets counts in breast cancer patients. Support Care Cancer 1999 May;7(3):149-53.

(109) Sanchez-Elsner T, Botella LM, Velasco B, Corbi A, Attisano L, Bernabeu C. Synergistic cooperation between hypoxia and transforming growth factor-beta pathways on human vascular endothelial growth factor gene expression. J Biol Chem 2001 Oct 19;276(42):38527-35.

(110) Schramm C, Protschka M, Kohler HH, Podlech J, Reddehase MJ, Schirmacher P, et al. Impairment of TGF-beta signaling in T cells increases susceptibility to experimental autoimmune hepatitis in mice. Am J Physiol Gastrointest Liver Physiol 2003 Mar;284(3):G525-G535.

(111) Schroth W, Goetz MP, Hamann U, Fasching PA, Schmidt M, Winter S, et al. Association between CYP2D6 polymorphisms and outcomes among women with early stage breast cancer treated with tamoxifen. JAMA 2009 Oct 7;302(13):1429-36.

(112) Selvaraj RK, Geiger TL. A kinetic and dynamic analysis of Foxp3 induced in T cells by TGF-beta. J Immunol 2007 Jul 15;179(2):11.

(113) Seton-Rogers SE, Lu Y, Hines LM, Koundinya M, LaBaer J, Muthuswamy SK, et al. Cooperation of the ErbB2 receptor and transforming growth factor beta in induction of migration and invasion in mammary epithelial cells. Proc Natl Acad Sci U S A 2004 Feb 3;101(5):1257-62.

(114) Shang Y, Hu X, DiRenzo J, Lazar MA, Brown M. Cofactor dynamics and sufficiency in estrogen receptor-regulated transcription. Cell 2000 Dec 8;103(6):843-52.

(115) Shevach EM. From vanilla to 28 flavors: multiple varieties of T regulatory cells.

Immunity 2006 Aug;25(2):195-201.

(116) Shimizu J, Yamazaki S, Sakaguchi S. Induction of tumor immunity by removing CD25+CD4+ T cells: a common basis between tumor immunity and autoimmunity. J Immunol 1999 Nov 15;163(10):5211-8.

(117) Shresta S, Pham CT, Thomas DA, Graubert TA, Ley TJ. How do cytotoxic lymphocytes kill their targets? Curr Opin Immunol 1998 Oct;10(5):581-7.

(118) Shull MM, Ormsby I, Kier AB, Pawlowski S, Diebold RJ, Yin M, et al. Targeted disruption of the mouse transforming growth factor-beta 1 gene results in multifocal inflammatory disease. Nature 1992 Oct 22;359(6397):693-9.

(119) Siegel PM, Massague J. Cytostatic and apoptotic actions of TGF-beta in homeostasis and cancer. Nat Rev Cancer 2003 Nov;3(11):807-21.

(120) Slamon DJ, Clark GM, Wong SG, Levin WJ, Ullrich A, McGuire WL. Human breast cancer: correlation of relapse and survival with amplification of the HER-2/neu oncogene. Science 1987 Jan 9;235(4785):177-82.

(121) Smyth MJ, Strobl SL, Young HA, Ortaldo JR, Ochoa AC. Regulation of lymphokine-activated killer activity and pore-forming protein gene expression in human peripheral blood CD8+ T lymphocytes. Inhibition by transforming growth factor-beta. J Immunol 1991 May 15;146(10):3289-97.

(122) Sporn MB, Roberts AB. Peptide growth factors are multifunctional. Nature 1988 Mar 17;332(6161):217-9.

(123) Suenaga R, Evans MJ, Mitamura K, Rider V, Abdou NI. Peripheral blood T cells and monocytes and B cell lines derived from patients with lupus express estrogen receptor transcripts similar to those of normal cells. J Rheumatol 1998 Jul;25(7):1305-12.

(124) Tai P, Wang J, Jin H, Song X, Yan J, Kang Y, et al. Induction of regulatory T cells by physiological level estrogen. J Cell Physiol 2008 Feb;214(2):456-64.

(125) Takeuchi M, Alard P, Streilein JW. TGF-beta promotes immune deviation by altering accessory signals of antigen-presenting cells. J Immunol 1998 Feb 15;160(4):1589-97.

(126) Thomas DA, Massague J. TGF-beta directly targets cytotoxic T cell functions during

tumor evasion of immune surveillance. Cancer Cell 2005 Nov;8(5):369-80.

(127) Thornton AM, Shevach EM. CD4+CD25+ immunoregulatory T cells suppress polyclonal T cell activation in vitro by inhibiting interleukin 2 production. J Exp Med 1998 Jul 20;188(2):287-96.

(128) Tobin SW, Douville K, Benbow U, Brinckerhoff CE, Memoli VA, Arrick BA. Consequences of altered TGF-beta expression and responsiveness in breast cancer: evidence for autocrine and paracrine effects. Oncogene 2002 Jan 3;21(1):108-18.

(129) Valverius EM, Walker-Jones D, Bates SE, Stampfer MR, Clark R, McCormick F, et al. Production of and responsiveness to transforming growth factor-beta in normal and oncogene-transformed human mammary epithelial cells. Cancer Res 1989 Nov 15;49(22):6269-74.

(130) van der Kuip H, Murdter TE, Sonnenberg M, McClellan M, Gutzeit S, Gerteis A, et al. Short term culture of breast cancer tissues to study the activity of the anticancer drug taxol in an intact tumor environment. BMC Cancer 2006;6:86.

(131) Veldhoen M, Hocking RJ, Atkins CJ, Locksley RM, Stockinger B. TGFbeta in the context of an inflammatory cytokine milieu supports de novo differentiation of IL-17-producing T cells. Immunity 2006 Feb;24(2):179-89.

(132) Vignali DA, Collison LW, Workman CJ. How regulatory T cells work. Nat Rev Immunol 2008 Jul;8(7):523-32.

(133) Wittke F, Hoffmann R, Buer J, Dallmann I, Oevermann K, Sel S, et al. Interleukin 10 (IL-10): an immunosuppressive factor and independent predictor in patients with metastatic renal cell carcinoma. Br J Cancer 1999 Mar;79(7-8):1182-4.

(134) Wrzesinski SH, Wan YY, Flavell RA. Transforming growth factor-beta and the immune response: implications for anticancer therapy. Clin Cancer Res 2007 Sep 15;13(18 Pt 1):5262-70.

(135) Wu WM, Suen JL, Lin BF, Chiang BL. Tamoxifen alleviates disease severity and decreases double negative T cells in autoimmune MRL-lpr/lpr mice. Immunology 2000 May;100(1):110-8.

(136) Xie W, Mertens JC, Reiss DJ, Rimm DL, Camp RL, Haffty BG, et al. Alterations of Smad signaling in human breast carcinoma are associated with poor outcome: a tissue microarray study. Cancer Res 2002 Jan 15;62(2):497-505.

(137) Xu J, Lamouille S, Derynck R. TGF-beta-induced epithelial to mesenchymal transition. Cell Res 2009 Feb;19(2):156-72.

(138) Yang YA, Tang B, Robinson G, Hennighausen L, Brodie SG, Deng CX, et al. Smad3 in the mammary epithelium has a nonredundant role in the induction of apoptosis, but not in the regulation of proliferation or differentiation by transforming growth factor-beta. Cell Growth Differ 2002 Mar;13(3):123-30.

(139) Yu Q, Stamenkovic I. Cell surface-localized matrix metalloproteinase-9 proteolytically activates TGF-beta and promotes tumor invasion and angiogenesis. Genes Dev 2000 Jan 15;14(2):163-76.

(140) Zheng SG, Wang J, Horwitz DA. Cutting edge: Foxp3+CD4+CD25+ regulatory T cells induced by IL-2 and TGF-beta are resistant to Th17 conversion by IL-6. J Immunol 2008 Jun 1;180(11):7112-6.

(141) Zou W. Regulatory T cells, tumour immunity and immunotherapy. Nat Rev Immunol 2006 Apr;6(4):295-307.

9 Danksagung

Herrn Prof. Dr. Cornelius Knabbe danke ich sowohl für die Möglichkeit auf diesem interessanten Feld zu promovieren, als auch für die stete Unterstützung und die Freiheit, die er mir während dieser Arbeit gewährt hat.

Herzlich bedanke ich mich bei Herrn Prof. Dr. Klaus Pfizenmaier für seine Bereitschaft die Arbeit von Seiten der Fakultät für Energie-, Verfahrens- und Biotechnik der Universität Stuttgart zu betreuen. Sein Interesse und sein Engagement haben mich sehr motiviert.

Herrn Prof. Dr. Matthias Schwab, dem Leiter des Institutes für klinische Pharmakologie (IKP), danke ich für die Möglichkeit diese Arbeit hier durchführen zu können.

Das Klima innerhalb der Arbeitsgruppe und unter den IKP-Kollegen im Ganzen habe ich stets genossen. Dr. Simone Popp, Dr. Matthias Stope, Stefanie Laukemann, Dr. Ina Abele und Dr. Heiko van der Kuip sei herzlich für die vielen Diskussionen und ihre Hilfe gedankt. Die Grundidee dieser Arbeit wurde freundlicherweise von Dr. Miriam Buck zur Verfügung gestellt.

Mein besonderer Dank gilt allen, die bei der Bereitstellung von Blut für die Immunzell-Isolierung beteiligt waren. Ohne das freundliche Entgegenkommen durch das Personal des Apherese-Labors im Robert-Bosch-Krankenhaus (RBK) wäre diese Arbeit nicht zu realisieren gewesen. An dieser Stelle seien vor allem Silke Brand und Dr. Beate Rothe genannt. Gleiches gilt für die Unterstützung bei den Versuchen mit primärem Tumorgewebe durch Prof. Dr. Wolfgang Simon und Dr. Andreas Gerteis aus der Gynäkologie, sowie Prof. Dr. Ott und Dr. Andreas Grabner von Pathologie-Abteilung des RBKs.

Der Robert Bosch Stiftung danke ich für die finanzielle Unterstützung während der Durchführung dieser Dissertation.

Ein großes Dankeschön geht an meine Eltern und die ganze Familie, die mir sehr am Herzen liegt. Vor allem danke ich Sabine Kohn für Rückhalt, Wärme und Inspiration.

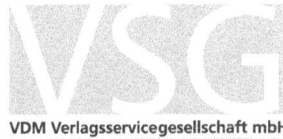

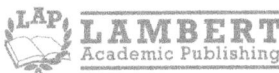

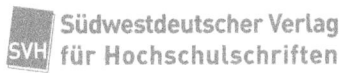

www.ingramcontent.com/pod-product-compliance
Lightning Source LLC
Chambersburg PA
CBHW021115210326
41598CB00017B/1452